Pocket Guide to
Culturally
Sensitive
Health Care

Barbara Stuart, RN, MSN
Catherine Cherry, RN, BSN
Jill Stuart, PhD

F. A. D

D0591802

Purchase additional ~~copies~~ ~~health~~
science bookstore ~~online at www.fadavis.com~~ or by calling 800-323-3555
(US) or 800-665-1148 (CAN)

F.A. Davis Company • Philadelphia

F. A. Davis Company
1915 Arch Street
Philadelphia, PA 19103
www.fadavis.com

Copyright © 2011 by F. A. Davis Company

Printed in China

Last digit indicates print number: 10 9 8 7 6 5 4 3 2 1

Publisher, Nursing: Robert G. Martone
Director of Content Development: Darlene D. Pedersen
Project Editor: Elizabeth Hart
Design and Illustration Manager: Carolyn O'Brien
Reviewers: Jeri L. Brandt, PhD, RN; Paulette A. Chaponniere, PhDc, MPH, BSN, BA; Stephen C. Hadwiger, PhD (Nursing), RN, Certified Parish Nurse; Joellen W. Hawkins, RN, WHNP-BC, PhD; Andrea Jennings-Sanders, DrPH; Janet R. Katz, PhD, RN; Cynthia Ploutz, RN, FNP-BC; Jean Rubino, EdD, RN, PMHCNS, BC; Hazel Sanderson, EdD, RN

As new scientific information becomes available through basic and clinical research, recommended treatments and drug therapies undergo changes. The author(s) and publisher have done everything possible to make this book accurate, up to date, and in accord with accepted standards at the time of publication. The author(s), editors, and publisher are not responsible for errors or omissions or for consequences from application of the book, and make no warranty, expressed or implied, in regard to the contents of the book. Any practice described in this book should be applied by the reader in accordance with professional standards of care used in regard to the unique circumstances that may apply in each situation. The reader is advised always to check product information (package inserts) for changes and new information regarding dose and contraindications before administering any drug. Caution is especially urged when using new or infrequently ordered drugs.

Acknowledgements

The authors are grateful to the following people for their reviews of individual chapters.

Bruno Ferraz do Souza, MD (Brazil)

Vivian Tong, PhD, RN, BC (China)

Danielle F Benjamin (Colombia)

Katherine Hirschfield, PhD (Cuba)

Naurio Tatis, MD (Dominican Republic)

Victor Fernandez, RN, BSN (El Salvador)

Kristina Bolten, BA, Cand. Med. (Germany)

Daphne Halikiopoulou, PhD (Greece)

Dan Egan, MD (Haiti)

Donna Marie Palakiko, MS, APRN (Hawaiians)

Mai Neng Lee-Xiong, RN (Hmong)

Arun Narayanasamy, RN, BA, MSc, M.Phil, PhD, DipN, FHEA (India)

Aaron Vicari (Italy)

Maxine Adegbola, PhD, RN (Jamaica)

Yamauchi Kyoko, MSN/MPH, FNP, ACNP (Japan)

Sung Ho Park, PhD (Korea)

Laura Robey, BSN, RN, MN, FNP (Mexico)

Aisha Abdallah-Joda, MBCHB (Nigeria)

Hifzah Tarik, BA, MSc (Pakistan)

Rose Constantino, PhD, JD, RN, FAAN, BSN, MN (The Philippines)

Anton Popov, PhD (Russia)

Abderrezak Bouchama, MD (Saudi Arabia)

Dr. Pauline Byakika-Kibwika (Uganda)

Connie Kim Yen Nguyen-Truong, BSN, RN, PCCN, PhD Candidate (Vietnam)

Debra K Thorson, MS, RN (Vietnam)

Due to privacy concerns, the reviewer of the Native Americans section requests to remain anonymous.

Contents

Cultural Health-Care Introduction

In 2008, the United States received around 38 million immigrants—double the number from 1980 and equivalent to 13% of the country's population. That is the equivalent of 104,000 immigrants per day; 4338 per hour, 72 persons per minute. Thus in 2008, on average, more than one person per second arrived in this country with the intention of living here—some of these immigrants enter legally, and some do not.

Many of these individuals likely have sought (or will seek) health care in the United States. Thus, health-care providers can benefit from a concise and targeted overview of the medically relevant cultural practices of these immigrant groups.

Health-care providers must be aware of pertinent cultural factors that affect health-care provision and decision making. Organizations with licensing authority agree. The Joint Commission on Accreditation of Healthcare Organizations notes on its Web site: "The Joint Commission is developing proposed accreditation requirements for hospitals to advance effective communication, cultural competence, and patient-centered care."

Even with limited effort, health-care providers can increase their knowledge, awareness, and sensitivity of cultural practices that are relevant to client care.

CONTENT OF THE BOOK

Because the patient population has changed to reflect a more integrated world, understanding some of the customs, preferences, and communication styles of others helps in providing safer, more personalized, interactions and will improve satisfaction levels for everyone involved.

Hence, the purpose of this book is to offer a basic foundation of cultural awareness in health-care workers. Perhaps this book will help with situations similar to those in the following true stories, gathered from conversations with people:

A couple originally from South Korea is in the maternity ward after the woman has delivered her first healthy child. The couple is astounded when ice cream and yogurt are delivered as part of the woman's first postnatal meal. Why? Many people from Korea believe that a woman should remain warm for up to 2 months after giving birth—including eating only warm foods and using extra blankets and clothes.

A family of Saudi Arabian heritage is strongly resistant to the idea of a near-death loved one being used for organ donation. Although there is no harm in asking the family if the patient is an organ donor, it can be useful to know that most Muslims from Saudi Arabia believe that the body should be buried intact and as soon as possible; the removal of organs or autopsy (and the time required to do such procedures) may be contrary to religious beliefs.

Consider the couple from Pakistan who come to the hospital for preterm labor. The physician makes the assessment, tells the couple what is best, then touches the woman's shoulder, saying, "We'll take care of you." A few minutes later, the woman reports that she needs to go to the bathroom, so the nurse leaves the room to give her some privacy. When the nurse returns, the couple is gone from the hospital and is now at high risk for delivery of a premature infant. Had the staff members been more culturally aware, they would have realized that in the Pakistani cultures, it is unacceptable for a man to touch a woman. The couple perceived as offensive what we would consider a reassuring tap by the physician.

STRUCTURE OF THE BOOK

This book provides information on cultural practices relating to 25 groups—from either the country of origin (e.g., Pakistan or Mexico) or an identified group (American Indian and Hmong). Twenty of the groups are recognized as having some of the largest numbers of immigrants to the United States. See, for example the Web site of the U.S. Census: http://www.dhs.gov/files/statistics/immigration.shtm. Four countries with large immigrant numbers in the United States are not covered in this book: Canada, the United Kingdom, Guatemala, and Poland; they were excluded due to a lack of sufficient information; however, future editions will try to include them. An attempt was made to include a country from all large geographic areas of the globe if there was reliable information and research available.

There is an exhaustive amount of information that the book could have included, but in order to make the book manageable size, we have included basic information in a number of categories. We strive to give health-care workers a taste of the type of information that they may find relevant in serving different cultures. If readers find that they are interacting with certain cultures on a more regular basis, the authors suggest learning about those particular cultures in a more in-depth manner.

The purpose of this book is to highlight possible differences between cultures, but it is also important not to generalize any specific information to all members of any culture. Individual assessment remains the best source of information. Many variables can alter patients' behavior or thought processes, such as knowledge of health, level of education, age, gender, acculturation, having a rural or urban upbringing, socioeconomic level, and feelings about being in a health-care setting. Immigrants take on and integrate American culture into their own lives in varying amounts.

This book is organized by cultures, and within each culture there are 11 subdivisions. These were chosen based on the majority of experiences that health-care workers have with patients.

- Communication
- Nutrition
- Physical illness
- Mental illness
- Pain

- Sexuality
- Childbearing
- Child rearing
- Family role
- Spirituality and beliefs
- Death and dying

Communication

Listed in this section are the primary and secondary languages for possible selection of an interpreter. This section covers eye contact and the extent to which it is expected and accepted. It also covers touching and whether, for example, shaking hands is a good idea. Questions answered in this section include: Do patients of this culture tend to be passive to the point that they agree with suggestions merely out of respect for authority but have no intention of complying? Is there a different manner of communicating with men than with women?

Nutrition

The nutrition portion covers which staples each culture prefers and what illnesses common to the culture may be nutrition-related. It discusses obesity as a by-product of nutritional habits. Questions covered in this section include: What do patients like to eat and drink? Which meal of the day is the largest? Are fluids better accepted hot or cold? Are there foods that are forbidden because of religious beliefs? Is being overweight considered healthy in this culture? Do people consume more fatty fried foods and avoid fruit? Is there a tendency for malnutrition or iron deficiency anemia?

Physical Illness

This section covers illnesses that may be more common to the culture as well as primary causes of death and physical injury. Questions covered focus on: Is this person from a country with high HIV/AIDS exposure? What conditions frighten these people the most? How is color assessed in a dark-skinned person? Are there concerns around bowel movements? Are there drug reactions unique to this population? Do these people take herbs that might react with their medications? Are some procedures, such as blood draws, particularly frightening to them?

Mental Illness

Mental illness is an area that some cultures disregard completely and others address directly. This section considers these questions: Is this a culture that acknowledges that mental illness exists as a biochemical imbalance? Does mental illness carry a stigma; if so, for the patient or for the entire family? Do these people believe that there has been some interference from a spirit to cause this illness? Do members of this culture accept therapy as a treatment for mental illness?

Pain

Everyone feels pain but everyone expresses it differently. One factor in knowing how a patient will express pain is culture. Various cultures also accept pain medications to different degrees. Questions in this section include: Is this a culture that expresses pain, or do members tend to suffer silently? Is there a difference in reaction between men and women? How do people of this culture feel about narcotics for pain? Do they have a preferred route for medications? Are there beliefs about pain being required for them to get better?

Sexuality

Sexuality is an area where cultures differ widely. Certain cultures accept extramarital affairs as part of daily life, whereas other cultures do not. This section also addresses questions such as: Are male children more cherished than female children? Are modesty and draping from the neck down of paramount importance? Are same-sex health-care providers necessary? How does the culture feel about homosexuals? Are AIDS and other sexually transmitted diseases acknowledged?

Childbearing

Childbearing is another area where cultures differ widely. It is important for health-care providers to know basics such as prenatal care and breastfeeding practices where there may be differences so that they can address the possibilities. Questions in this section include: Do people prefer a vaginal or cesarean birth? Are there beliefs about the quality of breast milk and appropriateness of nursing? Are dark spots on a baby's back a rash or mongolian spots? Does the father not want to attend the birth because he believes it is an intrusion into his wife's privacy?

Child Rearing

Childrearing is such a personal aspect of family life. There are, however, commonalities within cultures, such as the extent to which elders are respected by children and the value individuals place on education. Questions covered in this section are: Are there beliefs about weather that lead to bundling children with many thick layers? Are overweight children seen as healthy? Is physical discipline common, and what is the line between it and physical abuse? Does the culture believe in higher education? Is it available for both boys and girls? Is the culture more community- or individual-minded?

Family Role

The family role varies greatly between individual families as well as between cultures. Questions here include: Is the father or mother "in charge"? Are the children expected to stay close to home or encouraged to be independent from family? Will this be a family that will attend to all of the personal needs of the patient? How does the family care for the elderly? Does the family take in the elderly when they cannot live independently?

Spirituality and Beliefs

Religion and spirituality play a major role in how cultures approach health care, births, sickness, and dying. Health-care providers should be aware of religion as a factor when interfacing with all patients, not just patients of different cultures. This section focuses on questions, such as: What religions are prominent in the culture? Are there traditional healers, such as voodoo priests who may play a role in health and healing? Do certain numbers represent good and bad luck? Are patients likely to wear religious objects that they do not want removed?

Death and Dying

Another area where practices vary widely is death and dying. Topics such as organ donation and body preservation after death are worth considering. Some of the questions in this section include: Does the family not want the patient to know that there is a terminal diagnosis? Is this a culture that frowns on pulling life support? Is death a taboo subject? Do members of the culture prefer to die at home or at the hospital? Does a priest need to be called?

CONCLUSION

Across the United States every day, health-care workers interact with millions of people from immigrant backgrounds. This compact and easily accessible book provides the relevant materials on culture that are needed.

Health-care workers are privileged to be a part of their patients' lives at powerful moments, such as birth, death, serious illnesses, and emergencies. Being able to approach the care of patients and their families in a culturally informed way will potentially improve the experience. With knowledge of culture, health-care workers may also be more safety-conscious and improve outcomes.

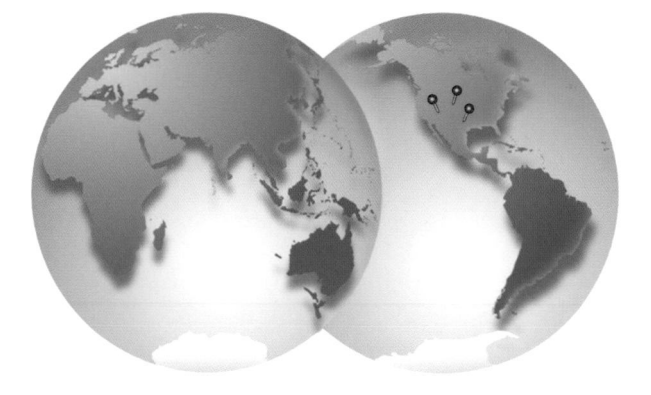

Native American

Native Americans, or American Indians, are the descendants of the indigenous peoples who inhabited the region known as North America. The native peoples of Hawaii, Alaska, and Canada are sometimes considered to be a part of this group. Their inclusion can be controversial in some circumstances because of the differences in the rights allotted to Native American tribes and Native Hawaiians and Alaskans. For purposes of this book, all Native American tribes are addressed together, keeping in mind that the different tribal groups of the United States often have very different cultures and beliefs.

The U.S. government recognizes 558 Native American tribes, and an additional 126 tribes are applying for federal recognition. Native Americans make up about 1.5% of the country's population, or about

4.1 million people. The states with the largest populations of Native Americans are California, Oklahoma, Arizona, Texas, and New Mexico. The Cherokee tribe is the largest, with over 300,000 people. The Navajo tribe is the second largest tribe, followed by Chippewa, Sioux, Choctaw, Pueblo, and Apache. Always maintaining their identities, many tribal groups have survived decades of troubles, including wars, forced moves to reservations, and plagues of diseases. Native Americans are still fighting many legal battles to recover, protect, and gain rights.

COMMUNICATION

- About 300 languages were spoken when North America was ruled by native tribes, and about 106 are still in use; however, many Native Americans speak English as well.
- Native American elders may not be able to read English well.
- The Sioux, Blackfoot, Cheyenne, and other plains tribes spoke a universal sign language, which is still in limited use today.
- People from many of the tribes avoid prolonged eye contact.
- Members of most tribes prefer larger personal space, and touching is not common.
- One family member may speak on behalf of the whole family.
- Many Native Americans, especially elders, prefer to communicate with someone of the same gender about health-care issues.
- Most Native Americans identify themselves as a member of a specific tribe, rather than generally as a Native American. Some strongly prefer the term American Indian to Native American.
- Listening and silence are appreciated in most of the tribal cultures.
- Speaking loudly is considered aggression in many of these cultures.
- Native Americans may use longer pauses in their speech between statements and are often interrupted due to this fact.
- Many groups are cautious with non-tribal health-care providers because of a long history of cultural conflicts.

- Most people are familiar with written consents and advance directives but may be hesitant to sign due to historical and present issues regarding the rights of Native Americans.
- Some believe that to speak about a disease or illness is to invite it into the body.
- In the Cherokee culture, it is considered polite to listen quietly to the person speaking, looking down, and generally not making eye contact until the speaker is finished talking.

NUTRITION
- Sharing food is very important in many tribal cultures, and patients may want to offer food to visiting relatives.
- Some cultures consider it impolite not to accept food that has been offered.
- The diet is typically high in fat, sugar and processed foods, which is very different from the traditional, healthier diet of most tribes.
- Corn is an important part of many traditional diets.
- Native Americans are reportedly four times more likely to not have enough food to eat.

PHYSICAL ILLNESS
- Accidents and violence are common causes of death and disability, especially in young males.
- Common causes of chronic health problems and death include heart disease, cirrhosis of the liver, gallbladder disease, and diabetes.
- Type II diabetes is a major problem in this population.
- Rates of different types of cancers are increasing in most populations, except for those living in the Southwestern United States, whose rates have remained low.
- Common types of cancer in this population include lung, colon and rectum, breast, prostate, cervix, stomach, pancreas, and gallbladder.

- Native Americans have the poorest cancer survival rates of all groups in the United States. This is thought to be related to a lack of access to health care as well as a cultural tendency to avoid pursuing health care for maintenance and even after symptoms are present.
- Many tribal languages do not have a specific word for cancer but instead use phrases such as "the disease for which there is no cure" and "the disease that eats the body."
- Native Americans and Alaskan Natives have the highest rates of smoking of any U.S. ethnic group.
- Some express problems with breathing as having a problem with the "air."
- People from this population are more likely to be obese, accounting for 30% of its population.
- Native American tribes generally accept Western medicine to treat illnesses but may also use traditional healers to further their treatment and healing.
- Traditional Native American healers may use herbs and other natural remedies that could potentially cause drug interactions.

MENTAL ILLNESS
- Native Americans have been found to have the highest rates of major depression of any U.S. ethnic group.
- They are 1½ times more likely to commit suicide than the national average. The Apache tribe has the highest rates of suicide.
- Alcoholism is a common illness in many tribes, largely the result of a genetic lack of an enzyme necessary for alcohol denaturing.
- Nearly 12% of deaths among Native Americans and Native Alaskans are alcohol-related, usually alcohol-induced motor vehicle accidents and cirrhosis.
- Drug abuse rates are also elevated in this population.
- Many tribal cultures believe mental health issues result from bad spirits.
- Many Native Americans will not seek or accept mental health treatment.

PAIN
- It is important to many Native Americans to remain stoic about pain.
- Members of some tribes use vague terms to describe their pain and may be able to express pain better by using pain scales or different signs and signals.

SEXUALITY
- Homosexuality was traditionally valued and embraced, but since colonization it has become controversial in many tribal communities.
- Men are traditionally the protectors of the family and the community; however, women are frequently the head of the family, making many of the family decisions.
- Women are three times more likely to be sexually abused or raped in their lifetime than the average American women.
- Women have low rates of abortion, which is thought to be at least in part the result of the fact that Indian Health Services do not provide for abortions.
- Cherokee Indians use several herbal types of birth control to prevent contraception.
- Many women are hesitant to use birth control because of a history of forced sterilization.
- Teenagers have the third highest rate of teen pregnancy of all U.S. minority groups, and its rate is increasing faster than in other groups.
- Premarital sex is common.

CHILDBEARING
- Mothers are three times more likely to receive inadequate prenatal care, or prenatal care not beginning until the third trimester.
- Because of biological issues predisposing Native Americans to alcoholism, fetal alcohol syndrome is more common in this culture.
- Some tribes believe that a pregnant mother should not tie a knot or braid as it may lead to problems in the umbilical cord.

- Some tribes have beliefs and practices regarding the placenta and umbilical cord of the newborn, such as burying or burning it.
- Infants may have mongolian spots.
- The Cherokee believe that for 3 months after birth, a mother should not prepare food for her husband or have intercourse with him.
- In the Cherokee culture a naming ceremony takes place in the first week after birth, at which time the baby is given a name.

CHILD REARING
- In some tribal cultures it is common for the grandparents to be the primary caregivers to the grandchildren.
- Parents often maintain an important role in their children's lives and choices long after the age of independence.
- Children are considered sacred in many tribal cultures.
- In the Navajo culture, girls undergo a coming-of-age ceremony called Kinaalda, when they become an adult.

FAMILY ROLE
- Many tribes were forced onto reservations with other tribes. This resulted in some long-standing battles between warring tribes that may exist today, and it also resulted in some families being of mixed tribal heritage.
- Many households are headed by a single parent.
- Families often teach their children about their tribal heritage and are very involved in their tribal community.

SPIRITUALITY AND BELIEFS
- Many Native Americans practice traditional tribal faiths involving a spiritual connection with nature. Some people may combine elements from their traditional tribal religion with other faiths, such as Christianity.

- Tribal religions may use feathers, crystals, or animal skins as symbols or objects of spirituality.
- Spiritual objects may be kept in pouches tied around the neck.
- Hair is important in many tribal cultures; cutting or losing hair is considered particularly significant.
- In the Navajo culture, chanting is an important practice for promoting healing and removing evil.

DEATH AND DYING

- Some tribal groups may not visit dying family members because they believe it is spiritually bad for the living and the dying.
- Some tribal groups believe it is important to keep feelings of grief hidden from the ill family member or friend and may appear happy and jovial around the patient. People close to the patient may express grief when the person is not present or has died, however.
- Different tribes have different cultural death rituals, which may include positioning the body, dressing the body, special places for funerals and burials, and burning herbs and grasses to purify the air.
- Organ donation is not widely practiced in many tribal groups.
- In the Cherokee culture the name of the deceased should not be said for 1 year after a death.
- In the Navajo culture, it is considered very bad for a person to die in the home.

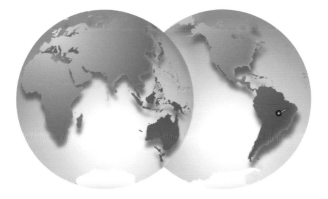

Brazil

The Federative Republic of Brazil is the fifth largest country in the world, both in size and population. Brazil is the world's fourth largest democracy and the tenth largest economy. The people of Brazil are primarily descended from the indigenous people who inhabited Brazil: the Portuguese explorers and settlers who colonized the area and the slaves who were brought in to provide much of the labor force for the new country. Brazil is also very multicultural, with the largest groups of Italians, Japanese, and Germans outside of their native countries. There is great income disparity in Brazil: much of the country's population lives in severe poverty, while an elite few boast great wealth.

COMMUNICATION

■ Portuguese is the primary language spoken in Brazil, although many
   Brazilians speak Spanish or English as a second language.

- Approximately 88% of Brazilians can read and write in their native language.
- There are more than 180 indigenous languages spoken in different parts of Brazil.
- Women from Brazil may greet people with a kiss on each cheek or a hug. Men generally shake hands with each other.
- Proper titles followed by a person's first name are appreciated in this culture and are used even within families; that is, John Smith would be Mr. John, or Marie Souza would be Mrs. Marie.
- Brazilians commonly use hand gestures when they speak.
- Brazilians place a great deal of value on friendly conversation and may consider it rude to rush through social interactions.
- Status is important and may influence communication, with greater respect being paid to people who are perceived to be of a higher social standing.
- In Brazil, it is considered obscene to make a circle with the fingers, as is used in the United States to signal "okay"; however, the "thumbs up" sign is likely to be understood.
- Brazilians may be comfortable with close personal space and physical contact.
- Brazilians may not adhere to strict standards of timeliness.

NUTRITION

- Approximately two of five people in Brazil have difficulty buying enough food.
- Many Brazilians avoid consuming cold food and drinks when they are ill.
- In some regions and among some generations, dairy products and fruits are thought to have negative effects when eaten together.
- Coffee is a popular drink that is consumed throughout the day.
- Brazilian cuisine varies by region, but generally meat, fish, fruit, rice, and beans are common.
- In some parts of Brazil, nearly 50% of children are anemic, and up to 12% have deficient vitamin A.

■ High levels of alcohol consumption—particularly among youths, especially young men—are sometimes attributed to tolerant attitudes about drunkenness.

PHYSICAL ILLNESS
■ The leading causes of death for Brazilian adults are heart disease and cerebrovascular disease.
■ In Brazil, accidents and acts of violence are another leading cause of death among adults.
■ Cancer is a common cause of death for the elderly and adults, with males more commonly being diagnosed with lung cancer, followed by stomach and prostate cancer. The most common cancers among women are breast, lung, and cervical.
■ Brazil had a large outbreak of dengue fever in 2008, primarily in the Rio de Janeiro area.
■ Brazil has one of the highest rates of leprosy in the world, although there has been recent success in improving levels of diagnosis and treatment.
■ Malaria is common in Brazilian communities near the Amazon rain forest.
■ It is a common practice in Brazil to bathe and wash the hair every day, even during severe illnesses.
■ Many medications do not require a prescription in Brazil, and family members may send medications to patients in other countries that they would not normally be able to obtain without a prescription.
■ Weight gain may be seen as a sign of improving health in this culture.
■ Physical appearance is also highly valued in this culture, and amphetamine-based weight loss drugs are commonly prescribed and, at times, overused.

MENTAL ILLNESS
■ Depression and anxiety are the most common mental illnesses reported in Brazil.

■ Brazilians may believe that medications to treat mental illnesses are addictive, and therefore those medications may be avoided or not taken properly.

■ People may avoid treatment for mental health problems, such as depression, due to the negative stigmas associated with mental illnesses.

■ Health-care provision for the mentally ill remains uneven in Brazil, although the country is generally regarded as being relatively proactive and innovative in its policies and programs.

■ Domestic violence is illegal in Brazil but remains underreported and problematic.

■ Many illegal drugs are produced and trafficked in Brazil, resulting in high rates of drug addiction, crime, and violence.

■ Brazil is the second largest consumer of cocaine in the world.

PAIN

■ Brazilians frequently report pain more readily than other populations and require more treatment for pain.

■ Brazilians often believe that over-the-counter or oral analgesics are not effective and prefer intravenous or intramuscular pain medications.

SEXUALITY

■ Despite being a predominantly Roman Catholic country, Brazil is known for its relaxed attitudes about sex and sexuality.

■ Although homosexuality is legal in Brazil, same-sex couples do not have the same rights as heterosexual couples.

■ Some social stigmas regarding homosexuality remain, particularly in rural populations; however, many Brazilian cities have strong gay subcultures.

■ Contraceptives are widely available in Brazil.

■ Despite the prevalence of birth control, teen pregnancy rates in Brazil have increased over the last 20 years.

- More women have tubal ligations in Brazil than in any other country in the world.
- Abortion is restricted in Brazil, except in circumstances of rapo or where the woman's life is at risk.
- Nevertheless, around one third of pregnancies are terminated in Brazil, and many of these torminations have complications and are performed illogally.

CHILDBEARING

- Perinatal complications are a common cause of death in Brazil, due to a lack of medical care for pregnant women in some parts of the country.
- Infant mortality is higher in Brazil than in many Latin American countries.
- Brazilian women may prefer cesarean deliveries based on a perception of their being more convenient; this may have contributed to Brazil having the highest rate of cesarean sections in the world, with nearly half of deliveries being cesarean.
- Brazil has experienced a rapid decline in fertility rates, falling from nearly 6 children per woman in the 1950s to 2.2 children per woman in 2008.
- The pregnant mother is encouraged to eat enough food for two people.

CHILD REARING

- The leading cause of death in very young Brazilian children is communicable disease (the most common of which are cholera, malaria, dengue fever, measles, tuberculosis, leprosy, and rubella).
- The most common causes of death of school-aged children are accidents and violence, followed by communicable diseases and cancer.
- Particularly in rural areas of Brazil, "bad winds" are sometimes thought to be responsible for making children ill.

■ "Evil eyes" or the bad wishes of an acquaintance are thought in some parts of Brazil to make children ill.

■ In traditional Brazilian families, male children are often given more freedoms than female children.

■ Disabled children in Brazil often remain at home and may not be integrated into society.

FAMILY ROLE

■ Brazilian families are often large and very close, and, particularly outside of urban areas, extended families frequently live together in one residence.

■ The family unit makes most medical decisions on behalf of the patient, who usually complies with the family's decisions.

■ Families from Brazil frequently will not leave the patient unattended by a member of the family.

■ In a traditional family, men are considered the head of the family, and the women fill the role of head of the household.

■ Women were declared legally equal to men in 1988, and there are equal numbers of men and women attending college and earning advanced degrees.

■ Brazilian families usually care for the elderly at home instead of utilizing nursing homes.

SPIRITUALITY AND BELIEFS

■ Brazil does not have a national religion, although 75% of the population claims to be Roman Catholic.

■ The large African slave population in Brazil combined its traditional beliefs with the Catholic faith to create new religions such as Macumba, Candomble, and Umbanda.

■ The indigenous people of Brazil practice many different tribal religions.

■ Amulets with the figure of a fist with the thumb between the first and middle fingers are believed to ward off bad spirits and to bring good luck.

- Ribbons are sometimes worn on the ankles, wrists, or neck to attract good luck; if possible, they should not be removed.
- Health promotion and screening may not be very familiar to some Brazilians.
- Traditional remedies may incorporate insects or parts of animals, using them, for example, in poultices or in mixtures for consumption.
- Physical attractiveness is extremely important in Brazil, and Brazil has more plastic surgeries per person than any other country in the world.

DEATH AND DYING

- In Brazil, family members often want to be told about the diagnosis before the patient is told, and the family may not wish to tell the patient about a poor prognosis.
- Hospice is frequently not acceptable to patients and families from Brazil as they see this as giving up hope.
- Cremation is becoming more common in Brazil, particularly as space for burial becomes more limited.
- Older generations may be very vocal in their grief, whereas younger generations are likely to be more reserved.
- Most Brazilian families prefer a rapid cremation or burial (within 24 hours); others may prefer a longer period of mourning, including a wake (taking up to a week).
- Autopsy and organ donation are not common practices in Brazil, although they may be more familiar to younger generations.

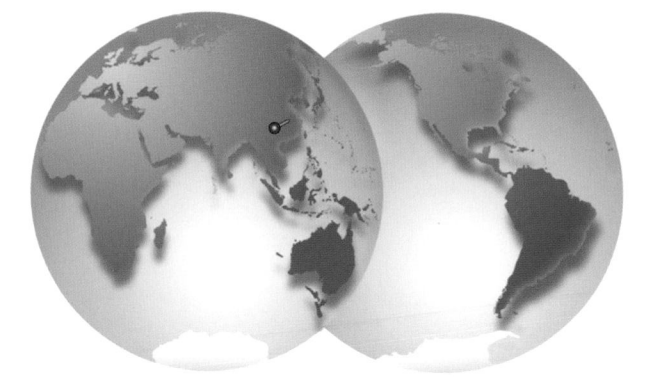

China

China is the most populated country in the world. Nearly 20% of the world's population, or one in five people, are Chinese. As of 2009, there were 1 billion, 330 million Chinese people. In 1979, the People's Republic of China, the ruling communist party, instituted a policy whereby couples living in urban communities can have only one child. Couples living in rural communities may have two children. Ethnic minorities are exempt from this ruling. In 2006, it was estimated that 1.2% of the U.S. population was Chinese or of Chinese descent, and this number is increasing.

COMMUNICATION

■ The primary languages are standard Chinese or Mandarin, Yue (Cantonese), Wu (Shanghainese), Minbei (Fuzhou), Minnan (Hokkien-Taiwanese), Xiang, Gan, Hakka, and a number of other minority languages.

- About 90% of people can read and write in their native language.
- A nod and a verbal greeting are considered appropriate; shaking hands or other physical contact is not common.
- Using proper titles such as Mr., Mrs., or Ms. is considered a sign of respect, and older people in particular generally prefer to be referred to by their proper title and last name.
- Children and young adults often address older individuals as "aunty" or "uncle" even though there is no direct family relationship.
- Direct eye contact is usually avoided with people who are perceived to be of higher or lower status, especially during greetings.
- The male head of the family may answer questions on behalf of the patient.
- Hand movements while speaking are not common and may be distracting to Chinese.
- Pointing and gesturing for a person to come forward is considered improper. The preferred way is to wave the hand in a cupped position.
- It is considered improper to touch one's mouth.
- People may be reluctant to ask questions, even when they are unsure.
- Saying "no" is frequently avoided as it is considered disrespectful, and people may not answer at all in order to avoid being disagreeable.
- When giving or receiving items, such as gifts, food, instruction sheets, or anything of value or importance, it is considered polite to pass the item using both hands.
- It is considered disrespectful to touch a person's head without permission; it should be done only when necessary because the soul is believed to reside in the head.
- Goods and services may need to be offered more than once as accepting things too quickly is considered impolite.
- Chinese may appreciate assistance from the care provider when discussing a diagnosis with family members.
- Winking is considered inappropriate.

■ Gifts are often refused three times before being accepted. It is considered polite to continue to offer repeatedly.

NUTRITION

■ Staples include rice, vegetables, seafood, and tofu.

■ Some food items are common that Westerners may be unaccustomed to, such as snake, cat, dog, carp, fish fins, turtle, and jellyfish.

■ The traditional diet often contains too much sodium.

■ In general, warm or hot water is preferred, and elders in particular prefer hot water.

■ Matching medications with certain foods and beverages is believed to yield maximum effectiveness and balance.

■ Rickets, which presents as very bowed legs, is common, especially in children living in rural areas. This results from a vitamin D deficiency, which causes low calcium levels.

■ Around 93% of people are lactose-intolerant.

■ "Asian flush" is caused by an enzyme deficiency. It produces a red flushed face when drinking alcohol.

■ Conditions associated with malnutrition, such as anemia, are common in parts of China, particularly in children.

■ Pica, common in this population, is the consumption of non-food materials, such as paste or dirt.

■ Foods, beverages, and medications produced in China may be contaminated or polluted because food and drug production are not closely regulated.

■ Tea is the primary beverage and is served at almost all social gatherings. Tea is believed to be beneficial to health.

■ Chopsticks are usually used instead of forks and spoons and should be offered when possible; foods served with chopsticks should be bite-sized.

■ Patients may believe that eating certain animal organs will repair their own corresponding organs.

- Burned rice tea is believed to treat diarrhea; however, serving a person burned rice is considered bad luck.
- Congee is a rice porridge often eaten for breakfast; congee is also believed to aid in recovery during illness.
- Using specific hot and cold liquids based on the nature of the illness is believed to bring the body's yin (cold) and yang (hot) back into balance, which achieves wellness. Most illnesses are "cold" illnesses and require "hot" foods and drinks. Rice is a neutral food; ginger is a yang food; and mung beans are a yin food.
- Dyspnea and vomiting are treated with hot soups and liquids.

PHYSICAL ILLNESS
- Cardiovascular disease is the most frequent cause of death, resulting from poor diet, lack of exercise, and smoking.
- Chronic obstructive pulmonary disease is the second most common cause of death because of high rates of smoking and the extremely poor air quality in most urban areas.
- Cancer of the lung, trachea, and bronchus are other major causes of death due to smoking rates and poor air quality.
- Cancer of the liver is another common problem, largely due to hepatitis B infections, which are often undiagnosed.
- Cancer of the stomach, esophageal, breast, and leukemia are other common types.
- China has the second largest population in the world infected with tuberculosis (TB). TB is often multi–drug-resistant and is often disseminated but found in less common sites, such as the bones.
- Many Chinese citizens receive a TB vaccine, called bacillus Calmette-Guérin vaccine, which causes the person to have a positive reaction to the purified protein derivative skin test for life and may leave a scar.
- Malaria, spread by mosquito bites, is common in the southern regions of China, and rates are noted to be increasing.

- Hand-foot-mouth disease (HFMD), which is different from foot and mouth disease, has infected more than a million people, mostly children, through fecal-oral routes and has caused many deaths. HFMD is caused by intestinal viruses and manifests as fever, blisters around the mouth, and rashes on the hands and feet.
- HIV and AIDS infection rates are estimated to be less than 1% of the population, but are increasing due to the lack of public health surveillance and public awareness.
- China has experienced outbreaks and fatal cases of sudden acute respiratory syndrome and avian (bird) flu in recent years, but they are not common diagnoses.
- Lead poisoning from toys, paint, the environment, and dinnerware is common, affects mainly children, and results in neurological symptoms.
- The skin tone of people of Chinese heritage varies greatly; caregivers should use caution when assessing pallor, jaundice, and inflammation.
- Patients may believe that blood draws will cause physical weakness and may therefore resist having this done.
- Ginseng is a common remedy and may be taken to treat anemia, colic, depression, indigestion, impotence, and rheumatism.
- PC-SPES is a combination of eight traditional Chinese herbs used to treat prostate cancer. PC-SPES contains estrogen and is not recommended by the U.S. Food and Drug Administration because use can lead to pulmonary embolisms.

MENTAL ILLNESS
- Anxiety, depression, and schizophrenia are the most common mental health illnesses.
- Psychotherapy is reserved for the seriously mentally ill and carries a social stigma.
- Depression is considered shameful and is not discussed openly.

- Suicide is prevalent and is one of the top five causes of death, especially in rural areas.
- Patients may benefit from smaller doses of haloperidol, an antipsychotic medication, and experience more extrapyramidal symptoms, such as extreme restlessness, involuntary movements, and tongue thrusting.
- Standard doses of antipsychotics, tricyclic antidepressants, and lithium may be related to serious cardiac changes.
- Gambling is very common and is on the rise due to the Internet. The Chinese government is attempting to reduce its frequency.

PAIN
- People may not readily express pain, but they generally agree to the use of pain medications.
- Offer pain medications frequently; patients may not accept them readily for fear of seeming impolite and may be ashamed or afraid to ask for them.
- People usually tolerate narcotics well, resulting in less respiratory depression and hypotension, but narcotics may cause increased nausea symptoms.
- Acupuncture and herbs are used to treat pain.
- Chronic untreated pain is common and is associated with higher rates of suicide, especially in rural communities where access to health care is limited.

SEXUALITY
- Modesty is very important and same-sex providers are preferred.
- Homosexuality is generally considered shameful and is illegal in China.
- People generally do not discuss sex openly.
- Divorce is not common; it is believed that as many as half of couples are not happily married.

- Marriages are sometimes arranged, especially in rural areas.
- Couples do not have sex during a woman's pregnancy.
- Abortion is sometimes used as a form of birth control, as are intrauterine devices and sterilization.
- Female reproductive issues are not discussed in the presence of males, even the patient's spouse.
- China has very high rates of abortion. This is due to the laws limiting child births and a strong gender preference for male children.
- Adult friends of the same sex may walk holding hands or arm in arm.

CHILDBEARING

- Urban couples are permitted to have one child, and rural couples may have two children.
- Ultrasound is often used to determine the gender of a fetus and may lead to abortion or abandonment if the baby is female. Males are often greatly preferred.
- Certain foods are believed to have negative effects when eaten during pregnancy: for example, bananas will cause the baby to have big ears, pineapple and shellfish will cause rough skin, and ginger may result in additional fingers.
- Men often will not attend the delivery, but female family members will.
- Women are frequently quiet and calm during labor and delivery.
- Vaginal delivery is often strongly preferred over cesarean section.
- Acupuncture is used to help with labor and delivery.
- Western medicines, including epidurals, are used to treat labor pain in more urban areas where there is more access to health care.
- Traditional Chinese cold foods, such as white gourds, are believed to be beneficial during labor, and warm liquids and warm foods such as mutton, should follow the delivery.
- It is believed that a new mother is *leurng* ("cool") and should be kept very warm. The infant should also be well bundled.
- Following birth, the new mother is often given ginger chicken rice wine soup to drink, which is believed to replenish the mother's

- blood and aid in lactation. The mother may also eat pig's feet cooked in a vinegar broth, which is believed to have a cleansing effect on the body.
- Fruits and vegetables are avoided following a birth as they are believed to weaken the body.
- During the first 100 days of life, the infant may be given chicken to eat as this is believed to bring good luck.
- The birth date of the child is extremely important due to beliefs about numbers and may influence the parent's behavior around the birth. For example, the number eight is considered lucky; a mother may try to encourage labor on the eighth day of the month.
- The traditional postpartum practice is called *zuo yuezi* ("doing the month"), during which time the woman and baby stay inside the home for at least 1 month and do not bathe or exercise. Staying inside has led to increased incidence of rickets in infants due to the lack of exposure to sunlight.
- At the end of the first month of the child's life, family members will have a party featuring red eggs and ginger to celebrate this milestone.
- The male head of the family typically responds to issues regarding the infant.
- Problems of the newborn are sometimes believed to be the result of bad things the mother ate or did during pregnancy.
- Newborn babies may have mongolian spots, which are blue-gray, blue-black, or brown, can vary in size and location, and may look like bruising. They typically disappear by age 3–5 years and should not be considered signs of child abuse. Some people believe that mongolian spots are the result of the gods having spanked the child in a former life.
- Circumcision of males is common.
- Neonatal jaundice is high in infants, with levels usually peaking on the fifth or sixth day of life.

■ The family may delay for weeks to months before naming the baby and may choose an "ugly" name to prevent spirits from wanting the baby.

■ Breastfeeding rates are about 60%–90% initially; however, infants are usually weaned at around 3 months.

CHILD REARING

■ Children attend school for an average of 11 years.

■ Due to the one child per couple rule, the" 4-2-1" problem has arisen, in which one child has two parents and four grandparents focused only on that child. This is also called the "little emperor" problem.

■ Sons may be treated as more important than daughters.

■ Children are potty-trained using split pants, which are split on the bottom and in the middle where the child passes waste. This practice typically results in rates of earlier potty training.

■ Because the soul is believed to exist in the head, it is believed that touching the head can be bad for the soul, especially in children whose soul is believed to be more fragile. It is preferable to obtain parental permission before touching a child's head.

■ Children who have difficulty in school may be a source of shame for the family. Teens and young adults who do not do well in school sometimes commit suicide because of the shame they feel for themselves and their family.

■ Children are often dressed in many layers of clothing because of a fear of cold. This can result in overheating and a delay in gross motor development due to the restriction of clothing.

FAMILY ROLE

■ There is a marked difference in family life and roles in rural and urban areas.

■ The family is considered more important than the individual.

■ Family members may take care of the patient's personal needs, such as bathing, instead of relying on hospital staff.

- Family structure is typically patriarchal, with a male head making decisions for everyone, or decisions may be left to the physician.
- The patient may have many frequent visitors; the family may believe the patient should never be left alone.
- Family members may wish to be informed of a bad diagnosis before the patient is told. The family may want to decide if it is in the best interest of the patient not to be informed about the diagnosis. This is a sensitive issue due to HIPAA regulations.

SPIRITUALITY AND BELIEFS

- About one third of people follow a religion. Common faiths include Buddhism, Taoism, Islam, and Christianity.
- The official religion of the People's Republic of China is atheism, because the cultural revolution promoted faith in the country as paramount.
- Exorcism may be used to drive out "evil spirits" that caused the person to become ill.
- Numbers have great significance. The number 4 is the unluckiest as the Chinese word for "four" sounds like the word for "death." Seven is also considered unlucky. The number 8 is the luckiest, followed by 6 and 2. Any number, from a room number or a floor in the hospital to the number of flowers in a bouquet, can be considered an indicator of fortune.
- Red is considered a lucky color, and pink and yellow are believed to represent happiness. Black, white, and blue are associated with death and funerals.
- Chinese astrology is a belief system that relates an animal to the year of birth.
- Illness is believed to result from an imbalance of the yin and yang, and patients may use herbs, acupuncture, diet, and various other traditional practices to restore balance.
- Cupping, which involves creating vacuum on the skin using heat (often fire) and a cup for drawing out the illness, may leave round bruises on the skin.

- Moxibustion, which is the practice of burning the herb mugwort on or near the skin to promote recovery, may cause scarring.
- Coining involves rubbing oil into the skin using a coin and may cause bruising or redness, which typically fades in a few days.
- Surgery may be avoided as it is believed to disrupt the life force energy *(chi)*.
- Good-luck articles worn on the body are considered very important, and patients are generally very resistant to remove them.

DEATH AND DYING

- Patients may believe it is important to remain alert up to the time of death, which may influence a decision about pain medications.
- Patients and family members may not feel comfortable discussing an upcoming death with anyone, including each other. Discussing death is believed to bring bad luck.
- Family members may want to bathe the patient after death.
- Three grains of rice may be placed on the tongue of the deceased to provide nourishment for the journey into the next life.
- Autopsy and organ donations are rare.
- Buddhist practices require a monk to remain with the body after death for up to 3 days in order to pray and guide the deceased person's spirit.
- Some Buddhists believe it is important not to show emotion near the deceased.
- Burial is more common than cremation, but cremation is common in areas where land is scarce.
- Elders may not show respect to younger people, so a child or a young adult will have a much smaller burial than someone older.
- Family members of the deceased may not visit friends for 30 to 100 days after the death as it is believed that the relatives of the recently deceased can bring bad luck into the homes of others.

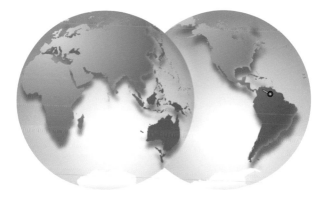

Colombia

The Republic of Colombia is located on the northwestern coast of South America. The country's population is estimated at around 45 million, composed primarily of people from three diverse origins: Ameridians, Europeans, and the descendants of African slaves. Approximately two million people of Colombian descent live in the United States. In the last half of the 20th century, Colombia was the site of prolonged armed political conflict between left-wing insurgents and right-wing paramilitary groups. Political instability and social unrest were exacerbated from the 1970s onward by Colombia's role as an international supplier of illegal drugs and the violent practices of the cartels that managed drug production and trade. Although many issues relating to the drug trade and political conflict persist, in the past decade there has been increased stability in many regions of Colombia. The stability is signified by dramatically lowered homicide and kidnapping rates and increased economic stability through production and trade in coffee, petroleum, coal, and cut flowers. Tourism is also on the rise as increasingly more visitors are attracted to the country's natural beauty.

COMMUNICATION
- Spanish is the national language.
- Around 80 indigenous languages are spoken; however, most people speak Spanish as well as their native language.
- People generally greet each other with a handshake. Women may grasp forearms instead of shaking hands.
- Proper titles are appreciated when addressing a Colombian.
- The distance for social interactions is less than 3 feet.
- Indirect communication is common. People may not answer a question directly but instead tell a story or talk around an answer. Being too direct may be considered impolite.
- Small talk is very important. People often feel more comfortable talking about health-care issues and share more information after talking with the provider about different conversational subjects.
- People may become very vocal and animated at times. This can sometimes be misconstrued as aggression.
- When Colombians feel comfortable with a person, they are open with their emotions and affectionate.

NUTRITION
- Colombians have a very diverse diet, incorporating a range of meats, fruits, breads, vegetables, and fish (in the coastal regions).
- Lunch is generally the main meal of the day; dinner may be eaten later in the evening than in the United States.
- Coffee (of which Colombia is a major world producer) is commonly consumed throughout the day.
- Alcohol is common, with beer being the most common, followed by hard alcohol, such as *aguardiente* and rum.

- Warm liquids (especially herbal teas) are believed to be beneficial for treating illnesses, and cold liquids are avoided.
- A hot drink made from sugar cane paste, called *agua de panela,* is a very common beverage and is believed to be beneficial in the treatment of respiratory infections.
- Protein deficiency and anemia are common, especially in children.
- Fast food is becoming more common.

PHYSICAL ILLNESS
- Although on the decline over the last decade, violence remains the leading cause of death, followed by cardiovascular disease, chronic obstructive pulmonary disease, diabetes, and cancer.
- Malaria affects about 15% of the population.
- Colombia and the United States have comparable rates of HIV at about 0.6%. People from Colombia with HIV are at increased risk of having tuberculosis.
- American trypanosomiasis, also known as Chagas' disease or South American sleeping sickness, is caused by a parasite commonly found in rural areas of Colombia. Symptoms vary depending on the stage of the disease. This disease is largely untreatable and can be fatal due to cardiac complications.
- Yellow and dengue fevers are common in the tropics.
- Many people sniff rubbing alcohol to relieve feelings of nausea.
- Bowel regularity is believed to be important for good health in many segments of the population.
- Exercise is believed to be unhealthy during illness, and patients may be resistant to ambulation and other physical activities.
- *Curanderos* are traditional Colombian healers; they use herbs, prayers, and massage.
- Physical beauty is considered important, and Colombia has more beauty pageants than any country in the world. Even prisons hold beauty pageants.

MENTAL ILLNESS
■ *Basuco* is an extremely addictive illegal drug and is made with cocaine powder. Its use is on the rise. Basuco powder may contain kerosene, gasoline, and sulfuric acid, and it often makes the user extremely paranoid.
■ One in 4 people have problems with anxiety, and approximately 1 in 10 have problems with alcoholism.
■ Mental illnesses are a major concern, but treatment is limited and unavailable for many; receiving treatment, however, is generally not considered taboo.
■ Domestic violence is a major problem.

PAIN
■ Men are less likely to express pain than women.
■ Most people believe that alternative treatments for pain, such as massage, heat, and ice, are acceptable and beneficial.
■ People generally prefer oral and IV routes for medications. Rectal routes are also generally tolerated.

SEXUALITY
■ Modesty is important, and same-sex care providers are preferred.
■ Men are three times more likely to have an affair than women, and infidelity may account for up to one-third of all separations between couples.
■ Same-sex partners have had many legal rights since 2007, although homosexuality remains taboo in many parts of Colombia.
■ Most women have tubal ligations, followed by the use of oral contraceptives as common birth control methods.
■ Colombia has high rates of abortions, which are illegal except under specific circumstances. These procedures are often performed improperly and frequently result in complications and death.
■ Premarital sex is very common; about 14% of teenage girls have sex before the age of 15 years.

- Teenage pregnancies account for around one in five pregnancies, and this rate is increasing.

CHILDBEARING
- Due to lack of available medical care, Colombia has high rates of infant and maternal mortality.
- The practice of having family members in the delivery room is a relatively new practice to people from Columbia, but it is generally well received.
- Children are typically given the father's last name followed by the mother's last name.
- Breastfeeding is more common in Colombia than in many other Latin American countries.
- Women may put cotton in their ears after giving birth to keep cold air out of the body.

CHILD REARING
- Public schools provide free education from first to fifth grades for approximately 5 hours a day, called primary studies. Any education children receive after primary studies must be paid.
- Children are protected and are taught to respect adults.
- Parents often teach their children to value religion, family, and hard work.
- An estimated 1.6 million children perform child labor.
- Colombia has the highest number of street children in the region after Brazil.
- More people are injured by land mines than in any other country in the world, with most victims being children.
- Colombia has large numbers of orphans living on the streets, primarily in major cities such as Bogotá. These children often perform illegal activities such as drug running, prostitution, and stealing to survive.

FAMILY ROLE

■ Colombia is a male-focused society, and the male head of family may make decisions on behalf of the other family members.

■ Elderly family members are often cared for at home; however, nursing homes are becoming more common. Many elderly also live in poverty because their family members have either died or abandoned them.

■ Families often focus a great deal of attention on ill members, which can sometimes interfere with plans of care.

■ Godparents (called *padrinos*) are chosen by the parents of a young child and play an important role in the person's life.

■ Catholic marriages have been legally able to end in divorce since 1991.

SPIRITUALITY AND BELIEFS

■ About 95% of people are Christian, with around 85% being Roman Catholic.

■ In the population, 60% of people state they do not actively practice their faith.

DEATH AND DYING

■ Family members often want to be told about the patient's diagnosis before the patient; the family may not wish to tell the patient about a poor diagnosis.

■ Colombia has created legislation that supports euthanasia for terminally ill patients in excessive pain or distress.

■ In keeping with the traditional Catholic faith, there may be a desire to perform last rights.

■ Organ donation and autopsy are often accepted practices.

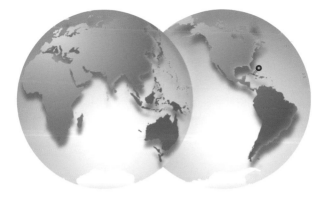

Cuba

The Republic of Cuba is an island country located in the Northern Caribbean. There are approximately 11 million people living on the island of Cuba, making it the most populous island in the Caribbean. At over 40,000 square miles, the island is the 17th largest in the world. Cuba became a Communist country in 1959 after a revolution brought President Fidel Castro to power. Cuba is the only socialist country in the Western Hemisphere. In 2008 Fidel Castro became ill, and his brother Raul took over the presidency.

Since 1962 the United States has held an embargo against Cuba, the terms of which have been revised several times. In the 1990s food and medications were added to the embargo list, although this has been moderated somewhat in recent years and is controlled by the U.S. government. While some political voices have called for an easing of America's restrictive policies regarding Cuba, others want the United States to maintain its posture in order to influence political change in Cuba. Many of these latter voices originate from within the Cuban-American population who want to see change in their homeland.

The 2008 U.S. Census found that more than 1.5 million respondents identified themselves as Cuban American, making this the third largest Hispanic group in the United States. Each year many more Cubans attempt to flee Cuba and emigrate illegally to the United States to escape poverty and political persecution. Despite its political and economic difficulties, the natural beauty of the island and friendliness of the people have earned Cuba the nickname of "Pearl of the Caribbean."

COMMUNICATION

■ The national language of Cuba is Spanish.

■ According to reports by the Cuban government 99.8% of people can read and write in their native language.

■ Eye contact is important when communicating.

■ Arguing is common and is not necessarily considered to reflect bad feelings.

■ People are sometimes thought to be outgoing and assertive in social interactions.

■ Women tend to be outspoken but may also hesitate to challenge male authority.

■ Immigrants who have left Cuba recently may avoid speaking directly about controversial issues and will use euphemisms and analogies.

■ In public, men are considered to be the head of the family and the decision makers, but women may in fact make most of the decisions within the home.

■ Close personal space is acceptable, and friendly touching is common.

■ People may not feel comfortable discussing certain subjects with people they do not know well, and initial efforts by a health-care provider to establish a basic level of trust may be appreciated.

■ People may ask not to be informed about health problems that have a poor prognosis.

- People may ask family and friends for advice before complying with the instructions of a medical professional.
- People may resist following medical advice that contradicts established cultural norms.
- Western medicine is generally valued and respected.

NUTRITION
- Rice and beans are diet staples, and meat as well as pork, chicken, and fish are preferred at all meals.
- Coffee is a popular beverage and is drunk throughout the day.
- Rum is a popular alcoholic beverage, especially during important social interactions.
- Hot and cold foods may be used therapeutically to treat specific illnesses.
- Food is very expensive and often accounts for a large portion of a family's budget.
- Food shortages have been a problem, and as a result, eating well carries cultural importance.
- Despite recent reports of some improvements in food provision, years of deprivation may make health messages about reducing salt, fat, and sugar unwelcome.
- Many traditional Cuban foods are fried in fat.
- Despite problems with food shortages, obesity rates are on the rise.
- Malnutrition in children was a longstanding problem, although reports from nongovernmental organizations suggest that this has been significantly improved in recent times.
- Physical exercise and sport are very popular with Cuban men but less common among women.

PHYSICAL ILLNESS
- An estimated 37% of adults smoke cigarettes, which most likely contributes to most of Cuba's major causes of death.
- Cardiovascular disease is the leading cause of death.

- Respiratory tract infections are the second leading cause of death and are statistically more fatal when they infect children.
- Cancer of the respiratory tract, involving the trachea, bronchus, and lungs, followed by chronic obstructive pulmonary disease, are the next most common causes of death.
- Prostate, rectal, and colon cancers are also major causes of death in Cuba and have also been linked to smoking, although not as directly as cancers of the respiratory tract.
- Suicide, violence, and homicide are together the fourth leading cause of death.
- According to government statistics, tropical diseases such as malaria, polio, and parasites have been reduced in recent years, but the accuracy of these statistics has been questioned.
- Nausea and vomiting are considered very serious symptoms.
- Pig skins are sometimes used on wounds like a dressing to promote healing.
- Followers of the religion of Santeria sometimes perform animal sacrifices to remove illness from a friend or family member. Some sacrifices involve rubbing the animal on the patient to transfer the sickness from the person to the animal.
- Bathing daily may be considered important, but wet hair is believed to exacerbate illnesses.
- There is a thriving black market economy that has developed due to shortages in the formal economy, and buying prescription medications illegally is common practice and carries no social stigma.
- Prescription medications purchased on the black market may be expired or have no Spanish-language instructions and as such may be taken incorrectly or inappropriately.
- Many people are unaware of the dangers associated with self-prescribing medications purchased on the black market.

MENTAL ILLNESS

- In recent decades, people with developmental delays, schizophrenia, and depression have been severely mistreated in the health-care system, which may discourage people from seeking professional treatment.
- Due to mistrust of health-care professionals, mental health issues are often addressed through informal networks, such as within families or through religious specialists.
- Many medications that are typically used to treat mental health disorders are not available in Cuba because of the U.S. trade embargo.
- Depression is often not well understood, and counseling and therapy may not be supported.
- Sedatives are a popular drug sold on the black market; many users are women.
- Drug abuse is severely punished in Cuba. This fact has resulted in generally low rates of drug abuse; however, in recent years cocaine use has been on the rise.
- Rates of alcoholism are high in this culture. It is estimated that up to 10% of people in this country may consume alcohol daily or regularly overconsume.
- According to recent data, suicide rates are around 20 men and 5 women per 100,000 people.

PAIN

- It is considered acceptable to express pain.
- Pain is treated in a variety of ways, including massage, relaxation, acupuncture, and music.

SEXUALITY

- Homosexuality is generally well tolerated in Cuba, especially in Havana.
- People who are residents of Cuba can receive sex reassignment surgery for free.

- Sexuality is relatively open in Cuba.
- The stress of small, crowded living space is thought to contribute to some extent to Cuba's having one of the highest divorce rates in Latin America; more than 60% of marriages end in divorce.
- Extramarital affairs for both men and women are more common in Cuba than in, for example, the United States.
- Contraceptives are provided free by the Cuban government.
- Teens often have sex as young as 14 years old; however, Cuba has low rates of teen parents due to sex education, contraceptives, and the availability of abortion.
- Abortion is legal and relatively common: approximately a third of pregnancies are terminated.
- Cuba has relatively low rates of HIV and sexually transmitted diseases.

CHILDBEARING
- It is believed in some parts of Cuba that pregnant women should avoid loud noises and looking at people with physical deformities because they can hurt the baby.
- The national birth rate is about 1.6 children per woman, which is leading to a decline in the Cuban population.
- Epidurals are not performed due to the lack of anesthesiologists.
- Fathers are not typically allowed in the delivery room. Other family members are also not usually allowed to attend a birth.
- Cuba's laws regarding paid maternity leave allows much more time than the United States.
- Infant mortality rates are lower than in the United States, although it is also more common to abort fetuses that indicate in utero abnormalities.
- Around 70% of infants are breastfed after birth, and nearly 50% are breastfed in combination with other supplements at 6–9 months.
- After the birth the baby's father may go out to celebrate with other men.

CHILD REARING

- Children attend school for an average of 16 years, with females attending an average of 17 years and males an average of 15 years.
- Physical punishment is generally considered an acceptable way to discipline children.
- Children commonly live at home until well after the age of independence. This reflects both financial and cultural reasons.
- Many parents place great value on their children's education.

FAMILY ROLE

- Family comes first for many Cubans, and most life decisions are made with the family in mind.
- Female family members will usually provide care for ill members, which extends to being present and offering care at the patient's bedside in the hospital.
- Elder family members are usually cared for at home and not in nursing homes or institutions.
- Frequent hurricanes and scarce building materials have contributed to severe housing shortages in Cuba. Multiple generations of families often share small dwellings, which may lead to strain on various family relationships.

SPIRITUALITY AND BELIEFS

- Cuba is officially an atheist communist country; however, about 60% of Cubans state their religion to be Catholic.
- Protestant denominations, which make up about 5% of the population, are viewed with some suspicion by the Cuban government.
- People may practice their faiths openly in Cuba, but the government does not allow religious schools or religious organizations to have their own media.
- Santeria is a religion combining Catholicism and the African religions of the country's early slave population and may be practiced in some form in Cuba by as much as 80% of the population.

- Some Santeria rituals involve human remains or other objects such as clothing scavenged from cemeteries.
- It is common in this culture to pin religious items to the patient's gown or bedding to help promote healing and protect the person.

DEATH AND DYING

- Patients and families often want to do everything possible to prolong life. As such, do-not-resuscitate orders are usually not accepted or signed.
- Santeria has many rituals associated with death and may include animal sacrifice. These sacrifices have been ruled illegal in a few American court cases, citing health and safety grounds.
- Death and dying frequently evoke responses of fear and sadness.
- Funerals are generally large ceremonies and often involve Catholic traditions, such as a wake.
- Cremation is very uncommon.

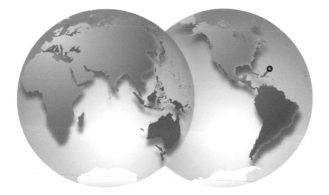

Dominican Republic

The Dominican Republic is an island nation in the Caribbean. The country is located on the eastern two thirds of the island of Hispaniola, along with the nation of Haiti. The Dominican Republic is the second largest country in the Caribbean, based on population and land mass, with around 10 million people and almost 19,000 square miles of land mass.

In 1492, Christopher Columbus landed on Hispaniola, and over the next 500 years the island experienced periods of governance by the Spanish and French, with interludes of independence and division, anarchy, and American intervention and occupation. During the colonial period, the indigenous population was decimated, and tens of thousands of African slaves were brought in, whose descendants form the main population of the country today.

Since the late 1970s, the Dominican Republic has been considered an independent representative democracy, with a presidential system similar to that of the United States. Sugar and tourism are two elements that contribute to what is, by some accounts, the second largest economy in the Caribbean. About 1.2 million Dominicans live in the United States.

COMMUNICATION
- Spanish is the primary language.
- Shaking hands is a common form of greeting for both men and women who are not well acquainted. Men who know one another may hug; women often greet other men and women with a kiss on the cheek.
- When approaching someone from this culture it is considered polite to say *saludos* to greet them.
- Proper titles, such as Mr. and Mrs. *(Señor and Señora)*, are appreciated in this culture.
- People are generally comfortable with direct eye contact.
- Communication tends to be somewhat informal, and people often talk openly.
- It is preferable to ask for permission before touching a patient.
- Written consents are not commonly used and may not be well received.
- Some people may speak louder and with more emotion than is common in other cultures.
- Some people, particularly those less educated, may be primarily focused on the present and not consider preventive medicine on a longer time-scale.

NUTRITION
- Traditional foods include rice and beans, seafood, potatoes, cheese, plantains and other fruits, and meat (chicken, pork, and beef).
- Foods that are fried and cooked in fats as well as fast food are common.

- Beverages and desserts high in sugar are popular.
- The largest meal of the day is usually lunch.
- Alcohol is commonly served at meals and gatherings, with beer and rum being two popular alcoholic beverages.
- Vitamin A, folic acid, and iron are common dietary deficiencies.
- About 9% of children suffer from growth retardation due to malnutrition.
- Hot and cold foods may be used therapeutically to treat specific illnesses.
- In some rural areas it is believed that pubescent girls should avoid eating fruits, particularly if those fruits have been warmed by the sun.
- Meal times may be considered social events when family members are expected to eat together.

PHYSICAL ILLNESS
- Cardiovascular disease is the leading cause of death.
- HIV and AIDS comprise the second leading cause of death, with an infection rate of 1.7%.
- Diabetes is another major cause of death but is often undiagnosed.
- Severe dehydration due to diarrheic process is a major cause of death among infants.
- Tuberculosis, along with other lower respiratory tract infections, is a major cause of death.
- Cirrhosis of the liver is a leading cause of death due to hepatitis infections and alcoholism.
- The use of acetaminophen as a popular medication for hangovers also potentially exacerbates liver problems in people from this population.
- Road traffic accidents are a major cause of death.
- The Dominican Republic has the highest rate of smoking of all the countries in Latin America, with roughly 65% of men and more than 25% of women being regular smokers.
- About 13% of men older than 15 years, and 18% of women, are obese.

- Skin care is important and may involve the use of oatmeal, yogurt, and oils on the skin, with frequent bathing.
- Some people believe that pouring cold water over the head helps to relieve dyspnea and breathing problems and helps revive people who have fainted.
- People are frequently not receptive to medications or treatments taken rectally.
- Exercise is not generally viewed as being important to good health.
- Particularly in rural areas, folk healers may be consulted before practitioners of Western medicine.
- Herbal pouches may be worn around the neck to assist the patient with recovery.

MENTAL ILLNESS

- Mental health problems carry a taboo. People with mental health disorders are often subject to discrimination.
- About 3% of men and 1% of women drink heavily daily, and 16% of men and 4% of women are periodic binge drinkers.
- The infrastructure for mental health is improving within the country; however, there is limited government support, and patients are treated only with their own or their family's permission.
- Suicide rates are high and are most often attributed to failed relationships.
- Particularly in rural areas, depression may be treated with herbal remedies and prayer.
- Prescription mental health medications are becoming available, particularly through private health-care providers.
- Anabolic steroids are legal. Men's use of steroids is believed to be relatively high.

PAIN

- People are generally comfortable expressing pain when asked.
- People generally accept pain medications.

SEXUALITY

■ Men may not respond truthfully about their health to female care providers in order to appear strong.

■ Sexuality is rarely discussed, even among family.

■ Homosexuality may be practiced in secrecy, and older generations in particular may believe that it is a curse, although younger generations may be more open about it.

■ Condom usage is low in some areas where sex education is minimal.

■ Menopause is not discussed, and men may think that once a woman has reached menopause she is no longer sexually appealing.

■ Abortion is illegal under all circumstances. Illegal abortions are often performed under unsafe circumstances and may result in permanent complications.

■ There is a relatively large sex industry, and adult prostitution is legal.

■ Female sex trade workers, many of whom are immigrants from other parts of the Caribbean (particularly Haiti) comprise a large portion of the HIV cases.

CHILDBEARING

■ The Dominican Republic has one of the higher rates of infant mortality for the region. This is believed to result from poor medical care in birthing units.

■ More than 90% of women received some form of prenatal care.

■ Complications from birth and pregnancy are the third leading cause of death.

■ Many people believe that cold liquids and cold night air can harm a developing fetus. Particularly in rural areas, it is believed that newborns and their mothers should avoid cold liquids and cold air for 40 days.

■ Bad news is thought to be able to harm a developing baby.

■ Many men believe it is an important sign of their masculinity to father sons.

- Frequently men do not attend the birth of their children, but female relatives are present.
- Laboring mothers may be very loud during delivery and frequently prefer the use of pain medications.
- The postpartum recovery period lasts for 40 days, during which time the mother is encouraged to stay in bed, and most of the newborn care is performed by female family members.
- Circumcision is not common.
- Breastfeeding is common, and some mothers may breastfeed their children for a few years.
- Particularly in more rural areas, infants may wear a charm made of black onyx to ward off "evil."

CHILD REARING

- In many traditional homes, female children are protected, and male children are encouraged to show their independence.
- Female children have a "coming out" at age 15 years.
- Male children are encouraged to become men and, in some families, be sexually active as teenagers.
- Playing baseball in the United States is a common goal for young men and may result in a great deal of pressure from their family; some young men even use steroids to improve their performance.

FAMILY ROLE

- Families are the strong social unit; most people are strongly tied to their country and family.
- Men are usually the head of the family, but single women are frequently the head of Dominican families living in the United States.
- Domestic violence is a problem but is often ignored.
- Daughters are expected to be the primary caregivers of elderly female relatives, and sons are expected to assist with the care of elderly male relatives being cared for at home.

SPIRITUALITY AND BELIEFS

■ Catholicism is the primary religion; Protestant churches have also grown rapidly in recent decades.

■ Many people do not attend services frequently but have an altar in their home where they worship.

■ People often strongly believe in miracles and the power of prayer.

■ Particularly in rural areas, traditional healers *(oungans)* are commonly consulted for spiritual healing.

■ Some traditional healers have been educated by Western medical professionals about how to recognize different medical conditions, such as HIV infection.

DEATH AND DYING

■ Many people prefer to die at home and usually welcome hospice care.

■ Death is not generally discussed, and family members often want to keep a bad diagnosis from an ill family member.

■ Organ donation is starting to become more common among family members.

■ Autopsy is not common but is acceptable if required by the family or official authorities in specific cases.

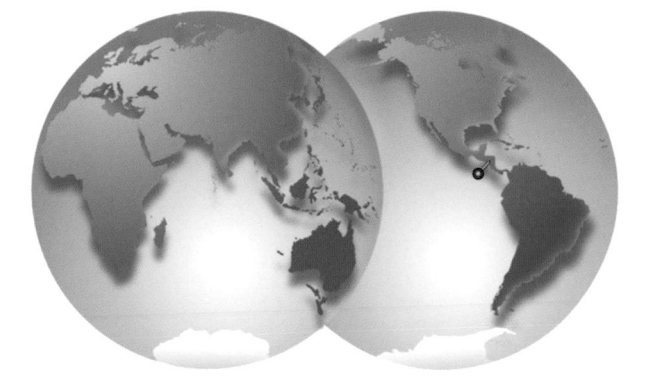

El Salvador

The Republic of El Salvador is a country located on the Pacific side of Central America. El Salvador has just over six million people, making it the 106th largest country in the world in terms of population. In encompassing only around 8000 square miles, however, it is both the smallest and most densely populated country in Central America.

El Salvador was occupied by indigenous peoples prior to colonization by the Spanish in the 1500s. In the 1820s the country began, along with other Central American countries, to achieve independence from Spain. The following century was characterized by periods of revolution and stability. A coup in the 1930s led to decades of oppressive and sometimes violent rule by military dictatorship. Most recently, the country endured a civil war that began in 1980 and ended in 1992. The end of the civil war coincided with social and economic reforms, which led to improved social conditions and international trade.

El Salvador has also endured frequent natural disasters. The country has been affected by recurring earthquakes and volcanic activity, as well as by occasional hurricanes, flooding, and droughts.

El Salvador is a democratic republic headed by a president. In the year 2000, El Salvador officially accepted the U.S. dollar as its form of currency. Money sent home from family members working in the United States is an important part of El Salvador's economy. Despite its many trials, the economy has been growing steadily since the mid-1990s.

COMMUNICATION

- The national language is Spanish. Some residents also speak an indigenous language but generally speak Spanish as well. English is also commonly spoken.
- About 80% of citizens can read and write in their native language; however, literacy rates in some rural areas are as low as 40%.
- Handshakes are an acceptable greeting, but women must extend their hand first for a man to shake. Some people may only nod when meeting others.
- People generally do not like loud speaking.
- During verbal exchanges to convey significant information, eye contact is important.
- Proper titles, such as Mr., Miss, or Mrs. are important. People are also addressed by their profession, such as Doctor or Professor.
- Pointing at people is considered rude.
- People tend to be very expressive with their hands and facial expressions during verbal communications.
- Yawning in public is considered impolite.

NUTRITION

- Traditional Salvadoran foods include *casamiento,* which is a mixture of rice and beans, tortillas filled with cheese or beans, fried plantains or yucca fruits, and other fruits and vegetables.

- The largest meal of the day is lunch.
- Coffee is a common beverage as well as thick drinks made from blue corn, seeds, and fruit.
- Fast food is becoming more common.
- About 19% of children younger than 5 years are chronically undernourished.
- About 11% of the total population is undernourished.
- Low protein intake, anemia, and deficiencies of riboflavin and vitamin A are common and can result in poor growth and development in children.
- Drinking water is often contaminated in rural and poor areas by runoff from agriculture, such as pesticides and fertilizers.

PHYSICAL ILLNESS
- Cardiovascular disease is the leading cause of death.
- Lower respiratory infections, primarily pneumonia, are the second leading cause of death.
- Violence and accidents, including traffic accidents, are also among the leading causes of death in this population. This is thought to have a relationship to high rates of alcohol consumption.
- Alcohol abuse disorders are the tenth leading cause of death, but most likely alcoholism plays a role in many of the other leading causes of death, including diabetes, cardiovascular disease, violence, accidents, etc.
- AIDS is another leading cause of death, but the rate of HIV infection is relatively low at 0.7%. Access to HIV medications is limited.
- Diabetes is a major cause of death due to the country's lack of available health care.
- Up to 80% of people are infected with parasites, one of the most common being Giardia. These parasites are often in the intestines and can cause chronic diarrhea, which can be fatal, especially in children.
- In the past decade, there have been outbreaks of dengue fever.

- Rural areas are known to have outbreaks of malaria, which has high rates of morbidity due to the lack of available health care.
- A few religious groups may be opposed to blood transfusions for religious reasons.
- Many types of medications can be purchased at a pharmacy without a prescription.
- Traditional healers *(curanderos)* are often consulted for treatment of physical illnesses.

MENTAL ILLNESS
- Alcoholism is a common problem.
- Suicide rates are relatively high.
- Due to El Salvador's high rates of national disasters, many people suffer from anxiety, increased stress, depression, and post-traumatic stress disorder.
- There are relatively few mental health professionals, leading to a large number of people with mental health issues being untreated.

PAIN
- Men are often stoic regarding pain.
- Women are often more expressive regarding pain.

SEXUALITY
- Women generally prefer a same-sex care provider.
- Families are generally patriarchal.
- Work places and public settings generally have more gender equality than home environments.
- Abortion is illegal, and women can be prosecuted for having one.
- Illegal abortions are practiced and often result in complications to the mother.
- Many women, especially in rural communities, marry between 15 and 19 years of age; however, many rural marriages are not official.

■ Official marriages performed in a church are considered irreversible.

■ Pregnancies before the age of 20 years are common.

■ There are no laws regarding homosexuality, but there have been reports of militia groups acting against homosexual people who were deemed "undesirables."

CHILDBEARING

■ Birth rates are among the lowest in Central America, at three infants born per woman.

■ Maternal and infant mortality related to childbirth is among the top 10 causes of death, due to the lack of access to health care.

■ Preterm birth accounts for 50% of neonatal deaths.

■ Neonatal complications are commonly caused by malnutrition and delayed growth.

■ Women who live in urban settings and work outside the home generally breastfeed for about 6 months, whereas women who live in more rural settings may breastfeed for up to 2 years.

■ Women often believe that eating chocolate, cheese, tortillas, and soup will encourage breast-milk production.

■ Up to 40 days after birth, women often wrap their heads and feet and put in earplugs to stop cold from entering their bodies.

CHILD REARING

■ Children attend school for an average of 12 years, but in rural areas 30% of children do not attend primary school.

■ Children may wear a red bracelet made from seeds to ward off the "evil eye" *(ojo)*, which is believed to cause illness and fevers.

■ An evil eye curse can be cured by chewing herbs, spitting them into a liquid, and then rubbing that liquid on the child.

■ Natural disasters may have affected the family lives of many children and caused them to develop a sense of insecurity regarding their safety.

- Older children are often expected to assist in raising their younger siblings.
- Malnutrition and intestinal parasites are a major problem and are often fatal for children.

FAMILY ROLE
- Extended family members are often close and support one another with raising their families, financially and emotionally.
- People may desire to attend to ill family members in the hospital as much as possible, staying close to them and even sleeping in their bed if it is allowed.
- Domestic violence is a significant problem.
- Young children are often raised by their grandparents and their older sisters.
- Women may be expected to play a larger role than men in child rearing.
- Nuclear families are the most common family unit; however, extended family homes and single-parent, especially single-mother, households are also common.

SPIRITUALITY AND BELIEFS
- About 51% of people are Catholic, and 21% are Protestant; 16% claim no religious affiliation.

DEATH AND DYING
- In the Catholic tradition in El Salvador, the night after a family member dies, the family will hold an all-night vigil. After the first night, family members mourn for an additional 9 nights of prayer.
- Organ donation is generally not well received, although autopsies are often allowed to determine a cause of death.

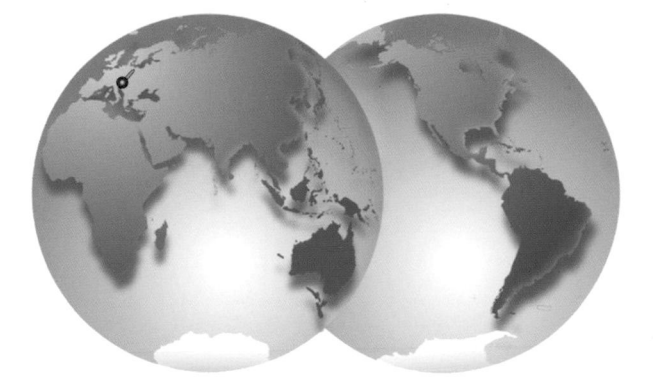

Germany

The Federal Republic of Germany is a European country with approximately 82 million people. In 1945, Germany was divided into two countries: the poorer, communist East Germany and the capitalist West Germany. Germany was reunified in 1990 with the fall of the Berlin Wall and the collapse of the Soviet Union. By the time the two countries became reunited, East Germany remained a relatively poor country, and West Germany had developed into one of the leading economies in the world. Unified Germany has, in the subsequent two decades, established itself as the fourth largest economy in the world.

Germany covers 138,000 square miles and is bordered by ten countries and two seas. Approximately 19% of Germany's population is of at least partial foreign descent, giving Germany the third largest immigrant population in the world. Germany has the fourth largest economy in the world, a very high quality of living, and a 99% literacy rate. In the 2000 U.S. Census, around 43 million Americans reported having pure or significant German heritage. This is the largest self-reported heritage group in the census, representing nearly 15% of the American population.

COMMUNICATION

- The national language of Germany is German, although it is not uncommon for people to be multilingual, and the younger generations often speak English.
- Handshakes are an acceptable greeting; it is considered rude to have the left hand in the pocket while shaking hands.
- It is appropriate to address people using proper titles, such as Miss, Mrs., and Mr.
- Direct eye contact is expected during communications.
- Physical contact, such as a pat on the back, is not generally welcomed in social situations, but it is usually considered acceptable in a medical examination.
- More than an arm's length of personal space is generally preferred.
- People tend to speak directly to the point and do not use a great deal of emotional inflection in their speech; they generally prefer that others do likewise.
- Chewing gum is considered rude.
- People tend to be very independent and have a particularly difficult time being dependent on others during times of illness.
- It is not a common German trait to be forthright with personal information and stories.
- People tend to be somewhat emotionally reserved.

NUTRITION

- Lunch is the main meal of the day, although breakfast is also considered important and tends to be fairly substantial.

- Traditional foods include sausages, potato pancakes, dense breads, and cabbage.
- The diet tends to be high in meat and fat, and foods are often cooked in lard; however, the younger generations are generally more aware of low-fat cooking alternatives.
- Recipes for cookies, cakes, and other sweets usually contain less sugar than American equivalents.
- Beer consumption per person is among the highest in the world, although public drunkenness is discouraged.
- Cold beverages are often preferred chilled without ice; hot tea or coffee is drunk throughout the day and, as a treat or snack, is accompanied by cake or a pastry.
- Due to high rates of alcohol intake, nutritional deficiencies are seen, especially in middle-aged males, because a large portion of their daily caloric intake is non-nutritive.

PHYSICAL ILLNESS

- The most common cause of death is cardiovascular disease.
- Cancer is the second most common cause of death, with trachea, bronchus, and lung among the most common types, most likely due to high rates of smoking.
- Colon, breast, and rectal cancers are also leading types of cancer.
- This country has the largest number of overweight people in Europe; a study in 2007 found that 75% of men and 59% of women were overweight.
- Germany has high rates of smoking, with more than 40% percent of men and 30% percent of women age 25–45 years being regular smokers.
- People may be very focused on regular bowel movements. Missing a bowel movement or an irregular appearance to a stool may be a source of great concern.

MENTAL ILLNESS

■ Alcoholism rates are high in Germany, with 1.7 million people in a country of 82 million people believed to be alcohol-dependent and needing treatment.

■ Drug abuse rates are on the rise; commonly abused drugs include heroin, hashish, and cocaine.

■ Because people tend not to express emotions readily, this may lead to dysfunctional relationship patterns and feelings of depression and anxiety.

■ Diagnosis and treatment of mental illness is increasing. This is particularly true of mental illnesses that are not severe in nature, such as anxiety disorders, which were previously often disregarded.

■ Mental health treatment tends to focus on the use of medications and not on psychotherapy.

■ Although acceptance and treatment of mental illness have become more common, mental health is still considered less serious than physical health.

PAIN

■ German patients may be stoic when in pain and hesitant to vocalize their discomfort.

■ There is a German saying that translates as "clenching one's teeth," which reflects the belief that one must endure until a situation improves.

■ Pain scales are a very effective way to communicate regarding pain due to a cultural tendency to be factual and specific.

■ People may be hesitant to accept pain medications without being provided information about the medication and its effects.

SEXUALITY

■ There is little significance placed on the gender of the health-care provider.

■ Wedding rings are worn on the right-hand ring finger.
■ Attitudes relating to premarital sex and birth control tend to be very open.
■ Germany has very low rates of teenage pregnancy.
■ Abortion is legal, but rates of abortions are very low.
■ Homosexuality is generally accepted.

CHILD BEARING
■ Breastfeeding is a common practice, and about 60% of mothers still breastfeed their infants at 6 months.
■ Pain medications are commonly used during deliveries.
■ Most women prefer to lie on their back during delivery.
■ About 30% of births are delivered by cesarean section.
■ In some faiths, it is believed that after a birth, the mother is considered impure until 6 weeks, at which time she is blessed by a prayer from the church.
■ With the exception of a small orthodox Jewish minority, the majority of German babies are not circumcised.

CHILD REARING
■ Students are divided into four secondary education groups, based on their abilities, interests, and future career plans.
■ Children on a college-preparatory path may not finish (the German equivalent of) high school until 19 or 20 years of age.
■ Children studying vocations may complete school by age 16.
■ Males must complete around a year of military or civil service, usually undertaken after completing (the German equivalent of) high school.
■ German parents may use logic and reasoning to guide the development of their children; many families have strict standards for their children.
■ Some parents have very high expectations for their children regarding education, career achievement, financial success, and so on.

FAMILY ROLE

■ Nuclear families are usually the primary family unit, and family members are generally treated as equals regardless of gender.

■ Two-parent households with one or two children are most common; German fertility rates are low, with an average of 1.35 births per woman.

■ Nonmarried cohabiting couples and children born out of wedlock have been on the increase over the last two decades.

■ About 30% of marriages end in divorce.

SPIRITUALITY AND BELIEFS

■ About 60% of Germans are Christians, with approximately half of those Protestant and the other half Catholic.

■ Approximately 2% of citizens state they are orthodox Christians.

■ The second largest religion is Islam, with about 5% of the population.

■ About 25% of people state they do not practice any faith.

■ German health-care practices are, for the most part, not influenced by religious beliefs.

DEATH AND DYING

■ People may be reserved in their expression of grief.

■ Family members or the patient may desire a visit from a religious figure (such as a priest or a pastor) in the final stages of life.

■ Do-not-resuscitate orders are understood and frequently accepted.

■ The majority of people die in nursing homes or hospitals.

■ Organ donation is not a common practice due to the complicated process involved; however, many people are open to the practice.

■ The body of the deceased is often brought home or to a funeral chapel for a viewing, followed by a funeral and burial or cremation.

■ A 3-day mourning period is practiced in many families.

■ Palliative and end-of-life care is not well understood, and only about 2% of people receive professional end-of-life care.

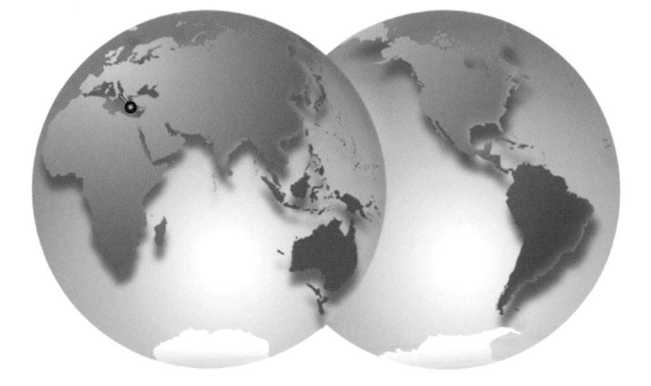

Greece

The Hellenic Empire (the official name of Greece) is a country in Southeast Europe, located on the Balkan Peninsula. Greece includes a number of islands in the Aegean Sea, making it about 51,000 square miles in area. The population is estimated to be more than 11 million people, which makes it the 76th most populated country in the world. About 10% of the population is composed of immigrants, half of whom are from Albania. Greece has its roots in the ancient civilization that originated around 1100 B.C. Greece is considered to be the birthplace of democracy and to have provided the foundation of Western civilizations. The country is a parliamentary republic and a member of the European Union. Between 1.5 and 3 million Americans claim Greek ancestry or have emigrated from Greece.

COMMUNICATION

■ The national language is Greek, and pupils learn English and one additional European language.

■ Around 96% of people can read and write in their native tongue, and many people can also read and write at least some English.

■ Handshakes are an appropriate greeting, and a kiss on each cheek is also a common form of greeting.

■ The father or oldest male is formally the head of the family, but female family members have very strong influence and should not be disregarded in decision making.

■ Close contact in personal space is acceptable.

■ Eye contact is an expected part of communication.

■ People tend to be quite emotionally expressive when communicating.

■ People may be distrustful of health-care providers and will look to people in the community for resources, information, and assistance.

■ It is common to visit several health-care providers before choosing one.

■ In this country patients often give physicians extra money to receive better care.

■ Families frequently believe that solitude is not beneficial and should be avoided, especially for an ill patient. Often, at least one family member will stay with the patient at all times.

NUTRITION

■ Common foods in the traditional diet include wine, cheese, breads, fresh Mediterranean vegetables, fruit, fish, and olives and olive oil. However, many of these foods are being passed over in favor of high-fat, sodium, and sugar alternatives, such as pizza, chips, ice cream, and fast foods.

■ Lunch and dinner are both considered important meals, with dinner usually eaten late in the evening, at about 9 p.m. or later.

- Milk is not commonly consumed beyond childhood and is often not digested well by adults.
- Coffee is very popular and is often consumed throughout the day.
- Chamomile tea is used to treat gastric upset, abdominal pain, colic, and menstrual cramps.
- Liquors are thought to help with sore throats and coughs.
- In households where orthodox faiths are practiced, people may not eat red meat on Wednesday and Friday.
- Wine is often served at meals.

PHYSICAL ILLNESS

- Cardiovascular disease is the primary cause of death.
- Cancer is the second leading cause of death, with tracheal, bronchial, lung, colon, and rectal cancers being the most common types, all of which are linked to high rates of smoking.
- Despite antismoking policies, around 40% of people smoke.
- Chronic obstructive pulmonary disease and upper respiratory tract infections are other major causes of death that are linked to high rates of smoking.
- Liver, breast, and stomach are other leading types of cancer.
- Two genetic conditions that are commonly diagnosed include thalassemia and G-6-PD (glucose-6-phosphate dehydrogenate).
- Obesity is a common problem, with 38% of women and 75% of men older than 30 years being obese or overweight.
- People commonly disregard physicians' orders, health and safety regulations, and health warnings, such as not smoking and wearing a seat belt.
- Traffic accidents are a major cause of death in this country, which is thought to be due to high rates of drinking and driving and failure to wear seat belts.

MENTAL ILLNESS
- Mental illnesses carry a social stigma and may lead to social isolation.
- Many people believe mental illnesses are inherited and may affect a person's bloodline.
- People often allow themselves to express anger, but anxiety and depression are often not shared.
- People frequently prefer treatment for mental health problems by medication instead of counseling.
- In the past decade, there has been more domestic abuse legislation so that abuse is generally considered taboo, and rates are decreasing.
- The rate of alcoholism may be as high as 40%; however, what is culturally defined as alcoholism may be different.
- Common illegal drugs include cannabis, cocaine, and heroin; overall abuse rates are believed to be similar to those of other regions of Europe.

PAIN
- Pain is believed to be a major indicator of illness and is thought to be a very bad sign that must be relieved quickly.
- The patient may be very vocal with suffering, and the family will often aggressively pursue pain medications on behalf of the patient.

SEXUALITY
- It is not uncommon for there to be little or no sex education at home.
- Birth control is generally accepted.
- Premarital sex is common and is largely accepted, particularly in urban areas.
- Rates of teen pregnancy are rising and account for over 10% of all pregnancies.
- Abortion is legal; Greece has one of the highest abortion rates in Europe.

■ Homosexuality is legal, but it is not considered acceptable in all groups.

■ Rape is significantly underreported and is often not severely punished when it is reported.

CHILDBEARING

■ People tend to have smaller families so they can better provide for their children.

■ Birth rates are very low, as with much of Europe, with 1.3 children per woman.

■ During pregnancy, food cravings are usually honored because satisfying them is believed to be best for the well-being of the baby.

■ About 98% of mothers receive prenatal care.

■ Fathers have not traditionally been present in the room during birth, but this is changing.

■ Breastfeeding rates are about 50% at 40 days after birth and 15% at 5 months.

■ People believe that mothers who take a shower too soon after birth cause the infants to have diarrhea and breast-milk intolerance.

■ New mothers are thought to be susceptible to illnesses and generally remain inside the home for 40 days after birth.

■ Family and friends coming to visit the newborn may leave silver coins and other objects inside the crib for luck.

CHILD REARING

■ Children generally attend school for 17 years before choosing a career or vocation or attending college.

■ Excess weight on babies is often considered healthy.

■ An estimated 40% of children from 9 to 18 years are overweight.

■ Type 2 diabetes in children is becoming more common due to obesity.

■ Families are often centered around the adults rather than the children.

■ Children are believed to be vulnerable to the "evil eye," which is a spell resulting from the envy of others. Symptoms are believed to include headache, chills, irritability, restlessness, and lethargy. Treatment is generally performed by the family matriarch or a healer and involves praying, making the sign of the cross, and putting olive oil and water on the afflicted person.

FAMILY ROLE
■ Divorce has been increasing over the last two decades, but at around 25%, the rate is lower than in many other parts of Europe.
■ The extended family is important but the nuclear family is generally considered the most important.
■ Fathers may portray themselves in public as the head of the family, whereas in fact the matriarch is often the decision maker.
■ Children often care for their aging parents and usually move them into their homes.
■ Reputation is generally very important to the whole family and may discourage some dangerous or risky behaviors.

SPIRITUALITY AND BELIEFS
■ Approximately 98% of people are Greek Orthodox Christians, and 1.5% are Islamic.
■ The Greek Orthodox church celebrates religious holidays on dates that differ from those of some other Christian churches.
■ People tend to be very superstitious and may also believe in miracles.
■ People may believe that sacrifice and suffering are honorable and may benefit others.
■ People believe that staring at, complimenting, or feeling envy of another person can make that person ill.

DEATH AND DYING
■ Families may wish to withhold a bad diagnosis from a patient until they believe the time is right.
■ People from older generations may avoid using the word "cancer" and refer to it instead as "the disease."

- After a death, the family may turn mirrors and photos toward the wall so that the spirit of the deceased may not be trapped in them.
- People may believe that dreams have significant meanings and that a deceased loved one is communicating with them in their dreams.
- Organ donation is not particularly common, but neither is it taboo.
- There are no particular stigmas relating to autopsy if there is a good reason for requiring it.
- Cremation has only been legal since 2006, and if deceased individuals have been cremated they may not have an Orthodox funeral.
- After death, there is often a wake at the family's home, followed by a funeral.
- Families may meet 40 days after the funeral to mark the end of the formal mourning period.

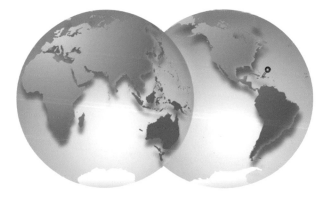

Haiti

The Republic of Haiti is an island nation in the Caribbean, located on the western part of the island of Hispaniola. The Dominican Republic occupies the eastern two-thirds of the island. Haiti is about 28,000 square miles in size and has a population of about 9 million people. Most residents of the country are the descendents of slaves who were brought to Haiti to work in the sugar fields after the region was established as a French colony. In the late 1800s, the slaves revolted, and Haiti became the only country to achieve independence through a slave revolt.

Since independence, Haiti has experienced periods of dictatorship, American intervention, and United Nations occupations of stabilization. The government is a semi-presidential republic, but Haiti still has an international reputation for corruption and human rights violations.

Haiti is one of the poorest countries in the Americas, with a low standard of living and whose people have a short life expectancy. In January 2010, a catastrophic earthquake devastated much of the island. Significant support from donors around the world was pledged; however, it has been difficult to translate that aid into long-term infrastructure development. There are an estimated 600,000 Haitians in the United States.

COMMUNICATION

- Almost all Haitians speak Haitian Creole; only around 20% speak French. French speakers tend to be better educated, wealthier, and have better job opportunities.
- About 53% of people can read and write in French Creole and/or French.
- Many people cannot read or write, so consents, instructions, and even medication names can be difficult. Some people may be embarrassed about this and try to cover up by pretending they understand.
- Due to low literacy rates, it is not uncommon to use pictures for Haitians to explain prescriptions, with images depicting morning, noon, and evening; and a space to mark how many pills to take at each time and for how many days.
- Shaking hands is an acceptable form of greeting.
- Personal space is usually about an arm's length of distance.
- People may be distrustful of interpreters, particularly if the interpreter speaks French and the patient speaks Creole. A Creole interpreter may be preferred by some Haitians.
- Physical contact is not well received in social settings.
- Eye contact is limited during communications, especially with people thought to be authority figures.
- Nodding the head may not actually indicate understanding or agreement, but rather just the desire to appear agreeable.
- When people communicate, they are often very expressive and may speak more loudly than other people.

- In Haiti, promptness is not as important as it is in some other countries, and people may not understand the requirement to be on time unless it is emphasized.
- People are likely to prefer frank and straightforward information.

NUTRITION
- People are often inflexible about their food choices and prefer to eat rice and beans with meat and stewed vegetables for their main meals.
- The largest meal of the day is lunch.
- Certain "hot" and "cold" foods are believed to promote recovery from certain illnesses that are thought to be "hot" and "cold" illnesses, which may not actually be related to temperature. For example, pregnancy is considered a "hot" condition and should be treated with "cold" foods, such as fruit.
- Around one in three people in Haiti does not have enough to eat.
- Malnutrition is a major problem in Haiti, with one-fourth of children being malnourished.
- Being overweight is considered a sign of health, which may cause people to disregard the negative effects of obesity.
- Fast food is becoming more common.
- Alcoholic beverages are common, including beer, rum, and a popular beverage called *clairin,* which is distilled from molasses.
- Eating garlic is believed to treat and prevent parasitic infections.

PHYSICAL ILLNESS
- Heart disease, cancer, and diabetes are three common causes of death.
- Common health problems include malaria, malnutrition and dietary deficiencies, hepatitis, and parasitic infections.
- There have been outbreaks of dengue fever and cholera in Haiti in recent years, including a serious outbreak of cholera in October 2010.

- In the earthquake, many people were seriously injured, including loss of limbs.
- In the earthquake, many people lost family members and their homes. Many people are still living in temporary housing (tent villages).
- After the earthquake, the lack of clean water and sanitation resulted in some outbreaks of disease.
- Hygiene is an important priority, especially during times of illness.
- People may be ashamed of vomiting and may try to cover it up.
- The use of oxygen is believed to indicate a very serious illness and may cause a great deal of distress for the patient and the family.
- It is sometimes difficult to obtain specimen samples as such body products are considered shameful.
- Many people believe that fatigue is simply the result of anemia and that it can usually be corrected by diet.
- The rate of HIV infection in this country is 2.2%, which makes it the country with the 28th highest percentage of people with HIV in the world.
- People may believe that illnesses are the result of spiritual causes, not physical ones.
- Men from this country have higher rates of tobacco and alcohol use than women, and rates are on the rise.
- Genetic defects seen in children may be attributed to spiritual influences on the mother and baby.
- Warmed castor oil is often rubbed onto the body of an ill person.
- People often believe that injected medications are the most effective form of treatment.
- Physical disabilities are often subject to social stigma and shame.

MENTAL ILLNESS
- Mental illnesses may be associated with shame and may prevent a patient from pursuing treatment or discussing symptoms.
- Mental illnesses are often attributed to supernatural causes and may therefore be treated with voodoo.

- People with acute mental health illnesses often become homeless or incarcerated.
- There is very limited treatment available for people with mental health problems.
- Since the 2010 earthquake, high rates of psychosis, anxiety, post-traumatic stress disorder, and depression have been reported.
- Haitians who lived through the earthquake may refer to it as "the thing" or "the day."
- People who emigrate from Haiti sometimes feel a great deal of guilt and depression about the family and friends they left behind and the poor quality of life they are living in Haiti.
- It is a common belief that fright is a serious condition that can be brought on by a bad event in a person's life and that it can lead to a stroke, loss of vision, and high blood pressure.
- People suffering from mental illness may describe their symptoms as headache, stomachache, muscle ache, and especially blurry or restricted vision.
- Rates of spousal abuse and child abuse are high. Women and children living in post-earthquake tent villages are particularly vulnerable to abuse.
- Abuse may be defined differently in this culture, where physical and sometimes violent discipline are considered acceptable.
- Much of the cocaine trade in the region is trafficked through Haiti; however, aside from small amounts of marijuana use, drug abuse is uncommon in this country.

PAIN

- People are often very vocal and expressive about their pain.
- People frequently do not understand the significance of the location and quality of their pain, which may make diagnosing health problems and treating their pain more complicated.
- Pain scales may be difficult due to high rates of illiteracy.
- People generally accept pain medications.

SEXUALITY
■ People may not discuss contraception, sexually transmitted diseases, or self-examinations due to feelings of shame about sexuality.
■ Contraception is generally not practiced because children are thought to be "gifts from God."
■ People generally wish to keep their bodies covered, even during medical care and treatments.
■ Premarital sex is generally forbidden for unmarried girls; however, it is considered more acceptable in rural areas. Males are generally allowed more sexual freedom as it makes them more "macho."
■ Abortion is legal only in cases where it will preserve the life of the mother; nevertheless, abortions are very common, are often practiced in an unsafe manner, and many women have permanent complications or die as a result.
■ The use of bedpans may not be well received, and patients may feel very strongly about getting to the bathroom and being able to close the door.
■ Many people believe nurses should be women and physicians should be men.
■ Homosexuality is mostly considered taboo.
■ Men sometimes have children with a mistress as well as with their wife.

CHILDBEARING
■ Women do not usually have access to prenatal care.
■ The average woman has just under four children.
■ Women may believe that during their pregnancy they should not swallow their saliva but instead spit it into a cup.
■ Women in labor may want to move around the room instead of remaining in bed.
■ Many women prefer not to use pain medications to help with labor pains.
■ Most women give birth at home without a skilled labor attendant.

- Some women may become extremely loud and excited during a delivery.
- Fathers generally do not attend the birth of their children as they feel this is a private matter.
- Many women may be resistant to having a cesarean section due to their fears about surgeries.
- Mothers often breastfeed, but they may be concerned about the "thickness" or nutritional quality of their milk.
- Women may take three baths with leaves in the water during the postpartum period. They may also drink the bath water as tea to promote recovery.
- After delivery the mother may wear a wrap or belt around her abdomen, which is thought to prevent the development of gas and to "tighten the bones."
- During the postpartum period, women often prefer warm or hot foods that are not white.
- Circumcision is not a common practice.

CHILD REARING

- Children may attend school for 12 years. Many children, especially in rural areas, do not attend school at all; less than 30% of children attend school to the sixth grade.
- Children of poor parents are sometimes given to wealthier families as servants and are sometimes abused in this situation.
- Infants and children may be treated with enemas, which are believed to remove toxins from the body.
- A child with diarrhea is considered to have a very serious problem. Diarrhea is sometimes believed to be brought on by a spell and is therefore treated by voodoo.
- Parents may delay seeking medical treatment for ill children because of lack of money and knowledge. Spiritual healing may be used instead.

■ What is believed to be acceptable physical punishment of children in Haiti is sometimes considered to be child abuse in the United States. Physical and even violent discipline is culturally acceptable in Haiti.

■ Infants and children have increased rates of umbilical hernias. Parents will often attempt to treat the hernia by using a coin or band to press on the protrusion.

■ A child's maternal grandmother may be the person responsible for the child's care. Since the 2010 earthquake, many women have taken on the care of many more children.

■ In some parts of Haiti, a man's status may be seen as enhanced by the number of children he has fathered.

FAMILY ROLE

■ Families are generally large, and officially the father is considered to be the head of the household. In reality, the mother is often the decision maker.

■ Men may have a second household with a mistress and children.

■ Divorce is becoming more common.

■ Since the 2010 earthquake, many children are orphans and live with neighbors or family friends.

■ Households run by single mothers are not uncommon, especially if the mother gives birth to a disabled child, which often leads to abandonment by the father.

■ The average life expectancy for people born before 2000 is around 50 years. Many families are unable to care for disabled elderly relatives, so many of the country's elderly are destitute and homeless.

SPIRITUALITY AND BELIEFS

■ 80% of Haitians are Catholic, and 16% are Protestant.

■ Voodoo is a belief system that is often practiced along with Christianity. It involves the worship of ancestors and protection from evil spirits and spells.

- People may believe in the "evil eye," which is the belief that envious or bad thoughts of another can cast a spell on someone and cause illness or other bad events to occur.
- It is commonly accepted that it is "God's will" that decides life and death, not Western medicine. Medical treatment or advice may be received with the statement "God willing."
- "Folk" medicine is followed by many Haitians. Where there is no interference, Western medical practices may be best explained as supplementary to traditional medicines.

DEATH AND DYING
- The oldest family member generally makes the arrangements and notifies the family members of a death.
- People generally prefer to die at home.
- Family members often travel great distances to be present after a death.
- Family and friends generally pray for 7 days after a person dies, followed by a gathering to honor the deceased.
- Family members often do all postmortem care.
- Many cemeteries were damaged during the 2010 earthquake, and the disruption of family members' burial plots has been distressing to many Haitians.
- Do-not-resuscitate orders and living wills are not common practices and are not generally well understood.
- Organ donation is generally not practiced because of the belief that the body needs to be intact for resurrection to be possible.
- Autopsies are considered acceptable, especially if the family fears that the patient has been turned into a zombie. The fear of zombies is common in parts of this country, especially rural areas, and is believed to result from a curse being placed on the deceased.
- Cremation is not common.

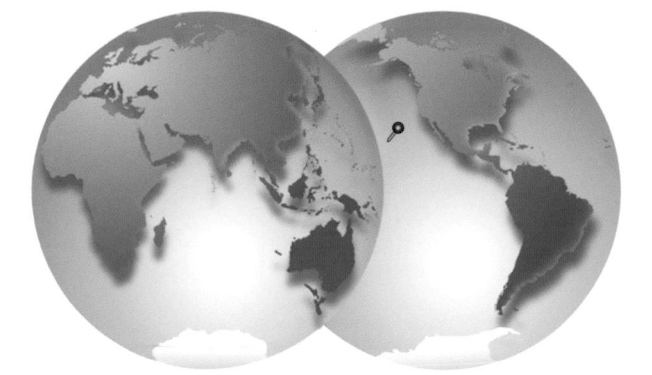

Native Hawaiians

Native Hawaiians are the descendants of the indigenous people of the islands, which became the state of Hawaii. It is believed that these indigenous peoples arrived on the Hawaiian Islands from the Marquesas Islands, Tahiti, Samoa, or possibly Tonga. The travelers are believed to have arrived as early as 400 A.D. The islands were separate, often warring, societies, until King Kamehameha was able to unite them, using new weapons and fighting techniques brought by the Brithish who arrived in 1778 with Captain Cook. With the arrival of Westerners came diseases, which spread through the islands and greatly diminished the Hawaiian population. The British continued to have a presence in Hawaii until the 1800s, when people from the United States began plantations and trading with the islands. In 1893, the United States overthrew the Hawaiian monarchy and officially made Hawaii a part of the United States. In 1959, Hawaii became the 50th state. Many people resent the fact that Hawaii is a part of the United States and believe that the islands should be allowed to become an independent nation again.

The state of Hawaii is a series of eight major islands in the Pacific Ocean. More than 400,000 people identify themselves as of Hawaiian or partial Hawaiian descent. Over 140,000 people identify themselves as pure Native Hawaiian. Native Hawaiians make up about 22% of the state's population. Many have moved outside the state and reside on the mainland United States and around the world.

COMMUNICATION

- Most Hawaiians speak English, but some also speak Hawaiian.
- The form of English commonly spoken on the Hawaiian Islands is called pidgin. Pidgin uses words such as *da* for "the" and *brudda* for "brother." Some Hawaiian words are also used when speaking pidgin, such as *pau,* which means "finished."
- Handshakes are a common greeting. Kissing on the cheek is a common greeting among close friends or as a formal acknowledgment.
- *Aloha* is a commonly used greeting: it means "hello," "love," and "good-bye."
- Native Hawaiians sometimes feel they have been subjugated by the United States and may be distrustful of outsiders.
- People often "talk story," which means to talk openly and casually. Talking story allows people to get to know one another and to gain understanding and information.
- Elder females are often referred to as "Auntie."
- Nodding the head may not indicate agreement but only that the person is hearing what is being said.
- *Mahalo* means "thank you" and is often said when two people are saying good-bye.

NUTRITION

- Common foods in the diet include rice, processed meats such as spam, barbecued meats, macaroni salad, and soda.
- The largest meal of the day is generally dinner.
- Fast food is very popular.
- The typical diet contains too much fat and sodium.
- The traditional Hawaiian diet consisted of fresh fruits, vegetables, fish, and products of the taro root. Many people are encouraging a return to this healthier way of eating.
- *Poi* is a paste made from the taro root and is a common food, especially during times of illness.
- A spam *musubi* is a popular food, which is a block of rice with a slab of spam on top wrapped in seaweed.
- Food is more expensive on the Hawaiian Islands because most foods must be shipped long distances, and this affects the quality of food some families can afford.
- Beer and other alcoholic beverages are often served at meals.
- Due to high rates of homelessness, poverty, and drug abuse, some Native Hawaiians may develop malnutrition.

PHYSICAL ILLNESS

- Native Hawaiians have a 44% higher mortality rate from cardiovascular disease than the U.S. population.
- Cancer is 39% more common in this population than in the U.S. population.
- Diabetes type 2 is a major problem because of high rates of obesity.
- Native Hawaiians are 21 times more likely to have tuberculosis than Caucasians.
- Native Hawaiians have a higher mortality rate from all health problems than does the U.S. population.
- Many people have increased respiratory problems due to *vog,* which is air pollution that rises from the volcano smoke.

- Dengue fever has not had an outbreak on the Hawaiian Islands since 1944; however, there have been several cases of dengue being imported to the islands in the last decade.
- Approximately 40% of Native Hawaiians are obese, as compared with 26% for the U.S. population.
- 32% of people smoke cigarettes.
- The *noni* plant is used to treat a variety of health problems, including bowel problems and menstrual cramps.
- Some Native Hawaiians do not believe in the effectiveness of Western medicine and may even believe that it is harmful.

MENTAL ILLNESS
- Addiction to ice, which is a form of methamphetamine, is a major problem.
- Native Hawaiians comprise about 28% of the state's homeless population, due in part to high rates of drug abuse.
- Spousal and child abuse is common but is often ignored.
- Native Hawaiians with drug abuse issues are less likely to have health insurance than people from other populations with drug abuse issues.
- The rate of alcoholism of Native Hawaiians is about equal to that of the U.S. population.
- Native Hawaiians comprise about 39% of inmates in this state.
- Mental health treatment, such as psychiatric medications and therapy, is generally accepted and practiced.
- One in five Native Hawaiians lives below the poverty line.

PAIN
- Some Native Hawaiians prefer to be stoic and not express their pain.
- Pain relievers are generally accepted.
- Alternative treatments for pain, such as massage, relaxation, and prayer, are accepted.

SEXUALITY

- Homosexuality is generally well tolerated.
- Birth control is generally accepted.
- Teenage mothers of Hawaiian descent make up 58% of the teenage mothers in the state.
- Women are usually the head of the family.
- Premarital sex is common, and about 36% of babies are born to unwed mothers.
- Abortions are practiced but are generally not discussed openly.
- About one in three Native Hawaiians never marry as compared with one in four Caucasians.
- People are less likely to be widowed, separated, or divorced than Caucasians.

CHILDBEARING

- Due to high rates of homelessness, drug abuse, and poverty, many pregnant Native Hawaiian women do not receive adequate prenatal care.
- People believe that wearing anything circular, such as necklaces or belts, will cause the umbilical cord to wrap around a fetus's neck.
- Fathers are often present in the delivery room and are helpful to the laboring mother.
- Some Native Hawaiian women believe that smoking ice before giving birth will help them to have an easier delivery.
- The rate of breastfeeding is nearly 90%; however, the breastfeeding rate among Native Hawaiians is 64%.
- Native Hawaiians who choose to breastfeed are significantly more likely to do so for a longer time than non-native Hawaiians.

CHILD REARING

- Asthma affects almost one in four Native Hawaiian children. This number is thought to be increased as a result of respiratory irritants such as increased mold resulting from high humidity and vog.

- Male Native Hawaiian children often are not circumcised.
- Children often live at home with their parents well into adulthood and may even raise their own children in their parents' home.
- Physical punishment of children is common.
- Native Hawaiian children are taught to value family, community, and, often, faith.

FAMILY ROLE

- *Ohana* is the Hawaiian word for "family," and it is an important theme in the Native Hawaiian culture.
- At least one family member generally stays with a patient during most of a hospitalization.
- Elders are generally cared for at home; institutional long-term care, like a nursing home, is usually a last resort.
- Grandparents often provide a significant amount of parenting of grandchildren.
- The cost of living is very high on the Hawaiian Islands, and families often have to work hard as well as pool their resources to maintain a good quality of life.
- Many families have become homeless due to the high cost of living. On the island of Oahu, there are large tent communities where some native people live on the beaches in tents and under plastic bags suspended in the bushes and trees, or they live in their cars.

SPIRITUALITY AND BELIEFS

- Many Native Hawaiians are Christian or Catholic and may combine aspects of the traditional Native Hawaiian religious beliefs with other faiths.
- The Native Hawaiian religion worshipped gods and goddesses, nature, and the human spirit.
- Illness is sometimes believed to be the result of a curse.
- A medicine man or Hawaiian healer is often consulted to heal the body and spirit.

DEATH AND DYING

■ Family members frequently stay with a dying member.

■ Native Hawaiians generally understand the concept of do-not-resuscitate orders and organ donation and may be open to these practices.

■ The *uwe* is a traditional Hawaiian death chant that involves wailing to express grief over the deceased.

■ Money is often given along with a card instead of flowers at a funeral.

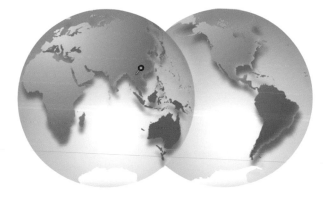

Hmong

Hmong (the H is silent; pronunciation is "mung") is an ethnic and cultural group that has lived in Asia for centuries. In most recent history the group has resided in the mountainous regions of Vietnam, Laos, Thailand, and China. There are approximately four to five million Hmong, with about three million living in China. The Hmong are sometimes called Miao due to inclusion in an ethnic classification created by the Chinese government. Hmong have lived in many parts of Asia but maintain a culture that is very distinct from other Asian cultures. During the Vietnam War, Hmong fought with U.S. soldiers against the Communist regime in Laos. Hmong were targeted by the government for their role in the fighting, and many fled to refugee camps in Thailand. The United States accepted many Hmong refugees as U.S. citizens and today there are an estimated 200,000–300,000 Hmong in the United States.

COMMUNICATION

■ Most Hmong speak a common language; however, many people speak the language of the country from which they emigrate. About 60% of Hmong living in the United States speak fluent English.

■ The Hmong language had no written form until the 1950s, when missionaries developed one, but it was never widely used by the Hmong people. Today many people cannot read and write in any language, including their own.

■ Shaking hands with brief eye contact is an acceptable form of greeting.

■ People may distrust translators who are unknown to them.

■ People generally prefer to speak to people of the same gender.

■ It is sometimes considered rude to begin to ask questions immediately after meeting a person.

■ People frequently say yes, even though they may not *agree* with what is said; saying yes is generally just an indication they comprehend *what* is said.

■ Maintaining self-respect is an important objective for people when they communicate; occasionally the meaning of what is said is lost in the interest of self-respect.

■ Pointing a finger is considered rude.

■ It is sometimes difficult to convince people of the benefits of Western medicine; however, gaining trust can increase patients' willingness to participate in their plans of care.

NUTRITION

■ Traditional Hmong foods include rice, vegetables, and fried or boiled meat.

■ Some Hmong believe that store-bought meat is not healthy and may eat animals that are grown at home.

■ Animal sacrifice is an important part of the culture, and the meat that is produced at such sacrifices is an important part of spiritual meals.

■ Rice and noodles are a major component of the diet.

- Dairy products and fruits are not a big part of the diet.
- Relatives of patients often bring food to the hospital because they worry the patient is not eating enough or eating well.
- People usually do not like ice in their beverages.
- Beer is the most commonly consumed alcoholic beverage.
- Alcohol is traditionally believed to have medicinal purposes.

PHYSICAL ILLNESS
- Some people refuse to discuss illnesses or problems that could have bad outcomes. They may even leave the hospital to avoid talking about such issues.
- Many Hmong believe that Western medicine can be dangerous and that it is designed for Westerners and is not safe for them.
- Health management and health promotion are not well received because the culture is focused on the present; less consideration is given to the future.
- Cardiovascular disease, diabetes, and kidney disease are common.
- Asthma and other respiratory diseases are common because of the chemical and biological warfare to which many Hmong have been exposed.
- More than half of Hmong adults living in the United States are overweight.
- People may be hesitant to report constipation as a health problem.
- Many Hmong have been exposed to contaminated foods and herbs from living in refugee camps and areas that have been the sites of wars and conflicts.
- People often expect medications to have an immediate effect that they can detect. If the effect is not immediate, patients often stop taking the medication after a couple of doses.
- Many patients do not accept any invasive procedures, even blood draws, and avoid seeking medical treatment if they fear this will become an issue.

- People often have strong beliefs that illnesses are the result of spiritual influences and that medical intervention is not beneficial or necessary.
- Some Hmong do not trust health-care providers and believe that the providers will use them for medical experimentation.
- Smoking is primarily for ceremonial purposes; the rate of regular smoking is lower than in the general population.

MENTAL ILLNESS
- The Hmong have endured wars and violence, have been refugees for many generations, and may suffer from post-traumatic stress disorder from such life experiences.
- Many Hmong have committed or attempted suicide as a result of being unable to endure their long history of hardships.
- People do not generally accept mental illness as a group of different diseases of the mind. It is often believed that the mentally ill person is communicating with different spiritual influences.
- Drug and alcohol abuse is relatively low.
- Some Hmong youths are involved in gangs, which are known to be involved in drug use and violence.
- Traditionally, mental illness is treated by an animal sacrifice, followed by a ceremony during which the animal is eaten, which is believed to remove the evil influences.

PAIN
- It is common not to express pain or communicate feelings of pain to anyone.
- Pain scales commonly used in hospitals may not be understood by Hmong people, especially because written communications are not common or well understood.
- Pain medications are generally accepted when offered, especially when provided with an explanation.

SEXUALITY

- Modesty is very important; same-sex providers are preferred, and it is important to keep the patient well covered.
- Homosexuality is not accepted.
- Many women do not trust hormone-based birth control as they fear it may make them infertile or ill.
- Many men do not tolerate wearing a condom.
- Many couples marry as young as their early teens.
- Premarital sex is common, and many marriages often occur when the woman first becomes pregnant.
- The Hmong often have marriage ceremonies that are not legally binding in the United States because they marry before the U.S. age of legality and because marriage can limit the government resources available to them as single parents.
- Abortion is not common.

CHILDBEARING

- Male children are preferred.
- Having many children is very important.
- Some women do not participate in prenatal care, especially invasive procedures such as pelvic examinations, unless they believe there is a problem.
- The father is often very helpful and involved in the births of his children.
- Some women prefer pain medications to help with labor.
- A shaman may tie an amulet or copper bracelet around a mother's abdomen to protect her from evil; the mother will most likely not want the bracelet removed during delivery.
- Women often do not want a cesarean section and may even avoid going to the hospital to avoid having one.
- The placenta is often buried at home so, according to belief, it can be located later by the person's spirit.
- Circumcision is not common.

■ Compliments to the newborn are believed to be dangerous as compliments call attention of the evil spirits to the baby.

CHILD REARING
■ Children are a very important part of the family unit.
■ The whole family participates in raising the children, including grandparents, parents, aunts, uncles, and older siblings.
■ Many parents dress their children to look like flowers so that "spirits" will not see the child but believe they are seeing a flower; consequently, the spirits will be tricked and prevented from taking the child to the spirit world.
■ The family unit makes all decisions for the children without any input from the children until they are considered grown.
■ Some people accept immunizations but have to be reminded to get them.
■ Teenagers are expected to help care for their siblings and may even have children of their own.

FAMILY ROLE
■ Families are often very large, and the oldest male family member is usually the head of the household.
■ The male head of the household often makes decisions for the whole family. Prominent male community members may also be consulted regarding major medical decisions.
■ Some families want to be informed about and consulted regarding every aspect of the patient's care.
■ Some families are polygamist; generally, all wives are of equal status. Hmong marriages are often not legally binding in the United States.
■ The daughter-in-law is expected to care for her husband's family, including his parents.
■ Elderly relatives are cared for at home.
■ Entire families often come to visit a hospitalized family member to provide care for them, including bathing and feeding the patient.

- Some marriages are arranged, and divorce is generally not accepted.
- A "bride-price" is paid to the bride's family at the time of a marriage.

SPIRITUALITY AND BELIEFS
- Many Hmong are Christian but combine the faith with practices from other religions, such as animism.
- It is a common practice to make animal sacrifices, especially to aid in healing.
- People believe that shamans communicate with the spirit world and can provide guidance toward spiritual healing.
- People often wear amulets and other religious jewelry, which they prefer not to remove.
- People often believe in reincarnation. This can affect a person's health or healing.
- Soul calling is a religious ritual during which a shaman calls the soul to return to the body.
- Some people may sew the parts of animals into their clothing and wear them to promote healing.

DEATH AND DYING
- The Hmong prefer not to discuss death and dying and will often refer to the terminally ill as just being tired.
- People do not discuss death with an ill person.
- Patients near death, or who have recently died, will often be dressed in multiple layers of their best clothing to prepare them for the spirit world.
- Buttons, zippers, jewelry, or any metal clothing fasteners cannot be on the body after death as this is believed to hamper the soul's ability to travel.
- People frequently believe that the bodies of the deceased should not be near one another as the souls may encounter one another and become confused.

- Organ donation is not often accepted as it is believed to affect reincarnation.
- Funerals must take place at a specific time so that the body of the deceased can be isolated from other bodies.
- Most people believe that death occurs at the time when the body stops breathing and do not understand the concept of brain death. This means many Hmong do not believe in stopping life support.

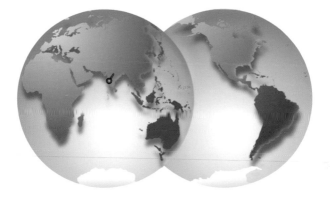

India

India is the second most populated country in the world, with close to 1.2 billion people. It is also the seventh largest country in the world by size, occupying most of a subcontinent that is over a million square miles. The history of civilization in this region dates back over 9000 years ago, when the first permanent settlement was developed. In the following centuries, the territory was ruled by numerous empires. From the 16th century onward, several European countries established trading posts in India, and by the mid-1800s Britain had formally established India as a colony.

India was a British colony until 1949, when Mahatma Gandhi led a nonviolent protest and India successfully gained its independence. At this time, Pakistan broke off from India and became a separate Muslim country. The two countries have been in a constant state of tension since, with both countries having developed nuclear weapons.

India is a parliamentary democracy and the largest democracy in the world by population. The country is divided into 28 states. These states operate under a federal government, but also independently and collectively they have a range of languages, religions, and cultures. About one-fourth of the people in India live below the poverty line; however, manyphysicians, nurses, teachers, and important scientists around the world have their family origins in India.

COMMUNICATION

- The primary language of India is Hindi, although there are 14 other official languages in India. Because of British colonization, English is commonly spoken.
- Roughly 73% of men and 48% of women can read and write in their native language.
- The proper way to greet a person is to hold the hands together in front of the chin and nod the head.
- Men may shake hands in greeting.
- Physical contact is generally limited.
- Nodding the head may mean "no," and shaking the head may mean "yes," which is the opposite of the practice in many Western cultures.
- People prefer personal space to be about 3 feet but will accept less room in crowded areas.
- Eye contact may be direct but not for a sustained time. Sustained eye contact with an older person or person in authority may be considered disrespectful.
- The caste system, in which there are defined levels of social classes, still operates, but this system is technically illegal and generally not discussed openly.
- Persons from the lower Indian castes in particular may be more submissive and deferential to health-care providers.
- Moving objects with a shoe or foot is considered rude.
- In India a gesture called the "head wobble" is common, and it has many meanings. Generally, it is used to acknowledge someone, to

- express agreement or sometimes disagreement, to communicate that the message is being heard, or to express friendship.
- Women may wear a red dot on their forehead, called a *bindi,* which in some regions of India signifies marriage and in some regions is worn for fashion and spirituality.
- Some people prefer the physician or other health-care provider to be the decision maker.
- The male head of the family may answer on behalf of the family, but the decisions are often made as a consensus.
- Older women, and especially the mother-in-law within a family, may have special status and be particularly influential in family decision making.
- People of older generations are held in high respect and may influence family decision making.

NUTRITION
- The diet is highly varied and may include rice, beans, chicken, nuts, fish, coconut, and vegetables.
- Many people of the Hindu faith are vegetarian. Many will not eat eggs, but they will eat dairy products.
- People often eat with the fingers of the right hand and are very conscientious about washing their hands before eating.
- It is considered polite in some parts of India to leave a small portion of food on the plate as an offering to loved ones who have died.
- There may be strict guidelines regarding who is allowed to prepare a person's food. This may result in family members bringing food to a hospitalized patient.
- Some families in India prioritize feeding adult male family members before females and children, which may result in malnutrition.
- Malnutrition is a major problem. Women and young girls in particular may suffer from protein malnutrition, thiamine deficiency, niacin deficiency, iron deficiency, vitamin A and B deficiency, and anemia.

- Lathyrism is a condition in India that arises from eating too many Lathyrus plants, which causes irreversible paralysis and muscle weakness. People consume this plant due to lack of other available foods.
- Conditions are believed to have "hot" and "cold" qualities, which are not necessarily related to temperature. For example, pregnancy is a "hot condition" and requires treatment with "cold" foods, such as fruits and vegetables, which may actually be served warm.
- About 15%–20% of people in India drink alcohol, with imported whisky being the most popular type of alcoholic beverage; however, alcohol is prohibited in some areas of the country.
- Being overweight may be seen as a sign of status.
- Eating black pepper and licorice is sometimes thought to protect a person's health.
- Water with cumin is believed to help with indigestion.

PHYSICAL ILLNESS
- The leading cause of death is cardiovascular disease.
- Conditions of the respiratory tract are major problems, with lower respiratory tract infections, chronic obstructive pulmonary disease, and tuberculosis being 3 of the top 10 causes of death.
- Some statistics note tuberculosis (TB) exposure rates being as high as one in two adults. TB is usually multi–drug-resistant in this population.
- Diarrheal diseases are a major cause of death, largely affecting children and people in rural areas and often caused by intestinal parasites, which are common.
- Traffic accidents are a major cause of death and injury in India.
- People have been exposed often to hazardous chemicals such as pesticides, pollution, and fertilizers because of poor water sanitation and environmental regulation.
- India has the fourth largest population of people living with HIV and the second highest death rate from HIV infection in the world. HIV/AIDS is another leading cause of death in this population.

- In recent years India has had problems with dengue fever and a disease that resembles viral dengue hemorrhagic fever called *chikungunya*.
- Bacterial meningitis is a major concern in India; it is spread through coughing, sneezing, and kissing.
- Outbreaks of viral avian flu and severe acute respiratory syndrome have occurred in recent years.
- Hepatitis A, B, C, and E are common infections in India.
- *Ayurveda* ("knowledge of life") is an Indian system of medicine that combines holistic medicine and natural remedies, along with spiritual and Western medicine.
- About 80% of people in India rely on herbal remedies.
- People may use many alternative remedies, including painting materials on their faces, wearing amulets, consulting astrologers, and applying poultices.

MENTAL ILLNESS
- Mental illnesses may carry strong social stigmas, particularly in rural areas where there is little available in terms of therapy or medications.
- Suicide is another leading cause of death.
- Although India's alcohol consumption rates are low relative to other countries, numbers are on the rise among younger generations, with the Indian government stating that just over 20% of men and 2% of women are regular drinkers.
- Drug abuse is also on the rise in younger generations, with cannabis, heroin, and illegal pharmaceutical medications being the most commonly abused.
- Because of social stigmas, patients may complain of physical symptoms instead of discussing their actual psychological complaints.
- People from lower castes are believed to have done bad things in their previous lives. This may lead to increased stress levels, depression, or a fatalistic attitude toward illness and treatment.

PAIN

- People may refuse pain medications due to fears regarding drug abuse and addiction.
- Pharmacological pain management and treatment are relatively new practices in parts of India.
- Hinduism teaches that suffering can be positive if it leads to spirituality. This teaching may lead to stoicism in its followers.

SEXUALITY

- Modesty is very important, and same-sex providers are often preferred.
- Homosexuality is generally not accepted or even discussed in parts of India, although in some areas eunuchs (castrated males) and male cross-dressers are considered a part of local culture.
- Marriages are often arranged.
- Divorce may not be an option or may not be recognized in some regions of India.
- In some parts of India the husband may take a second wife if the first wife is believed to be infertile.
- In northern India, women may cover their body and their face with a veil.
- A Hindu or Muslim woman who is menstruating may not be allowed to cook or attend prayers.
- Women in India have varying amounts of freedom based on the family to which they belong or marry into and the area in which they live.
- Women are often hesitant about taking oral contraceptives and prefer intrauterine devices, condoms, withdrawal, and the rhythm method. Sterilization is also an accepted practice in India.
- Marrying as young as 15–19 years old and having children is a common practice, usually in more rural parts of India.
- Abortions are legal in India, but they are often performed in unhygienic and unsafe facilities.

- In India it is common for a fetus to be aborted after discovering it is female, but in recent years this practice has become illegal.

CHILDBEARING
- Being pregnant increases the status of a woman.
- Many laboring women are not managed by a skilled birthing attendant, causing rates of perinatal complications to be among the leading causes of death.
- It is believed that women should be quiet and stoic during delivery.
- Pain relievers are generally not used during deliveries in India because they are thought to cause complications.
- Men are generally not present in the delivery room; instead, a female family member will attend the birth.
- The sex of the infant may not be announced until the placenta is delivered.
- After a birth, there is generally a female caregiver or family member who provides most of the care of the family, mother and newborn being given 40 days of rest.
- Colostrum is believed to be unhealthy for the baby; however, breast-feeding is accepted and may be done for 6 months and up to 3 years.
- Breastfeeding babies are often supplemented with cow's milk diluted with sugar water as this is thought to be gentle on a newborn's stomach.
- After childbirth, the mother is believed to need "hot" foods, such as a bread dish called *katlu* or *panjiri,* dried fish, drumsticks, and greens, to keep her body warm physically. This practice is also believed to increase lactation.
- A ritual called the sixth may be practiced on the 6th day of life. It involves rubbing red paste onto the palms and soles of the infant and welcoming the Holy Spirit into them.
- A baby may be officially named on the 11th day of life during what is called the cradle ritual, in which ceremonies are practiced to protect the baby from evil spirits.

CHILD REARING

- The average child attends school for 10 years.
- Parenting generally involves the whole family, including grandparents, and children may be as attached to their grandparents as they are to their parents.
- Children may sleep with their parents from infancy until early childhood.
- Most children are raised to respect their elders, honor their family, and maintain their moral values.
- In some sections of Indian society children are raised to value their education highly. The pressure is sometimes emphasized to the point that children suffer extreme stress and depression regarding their education.
- Because of gender issues, sometimes only male children are given proper health care, including immunizations.
- Children are seldom praised because of the risk of calling attention to them and bringing an "evil eye" on them.
- Children are often given many duties and chores at a younger age to teach them responsibility.

FAMILY ROLE

- It is common for the extended family to live in a single home, including grandparents, parents, children, and even uncles and their families.
- In India, the youngest son is expected to care for his parents in their retirement years.
- Men are usually the head of the household, and older family members have more status than younger family members in India. Nonetheless, important family decisions, such as health-care issues, are often reached through family consensus.
- In parts of this country, spousal abuse is considered to be a private matter between the husband and wife.
- Arranged marriages of teenage girls are common in some rural parts of India.

SPIRITUALITY AND BELIEFS

- The people of India are 80% Hindu, 13% Muslim, and 2% Christian.
- Even among Indian Hindus there are differences in spiritual practices.
- Sikhs are a religious group in India who share some beliefs with the Hindu faith but worship only one deity and do not believe in cutting the hair.
- Hindus and Muslims have special religious dietary considerations.
- *Ayurveda* requires that the five elements of earth, water, fire, air and ether be in balance. Believers achieve balance through yoga, meditation, chanting, and rhythmic breathing.
- Hindus normally remove their shoes to enter holy places.

DEATH AND DYING

- The family of a patient may want to be told about a bad prognosis before the patient is told.
- Death is often met with acceptance in the Indian culture because, with the belief in reincarnation, the person is merely passing to another life.
- Many followers of the Hindu faith prefer to die at home or may even return to India to die, if possible.
- The body is usually washed by a family member and wrapped in a red cloth after death.
- Some Hindus believe it is important to put water from the Ganges River into the mouth of the dying person.
- Cremation is more common than burial in India.
- Organ donation and autopsy are not common.

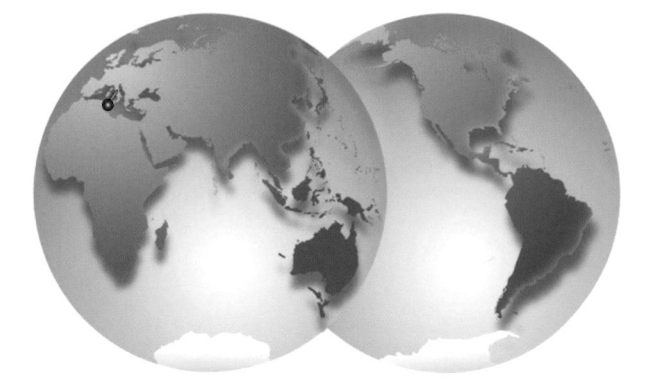

Italy

The Italian Republic is located in southern Europe on the Italian peninsula. Italy has 60 million inhabitants, making it the 23rd most populated country in the world. The capital city is Rome, which was once the heart of the Roman Empire. The Roman Empire existed from approximately 20 B.C. to 500 A.D., during which time it was a center of Western cultural, political, religious, and scientific importance. The headquarters of the Catholic Church is located within Rome, as an independent city-state named Vatican City (population approximately 800). Italy is approximately 116,400 square miles and is a democratic republic headed by a president.

COMMUNICATION

■ Italian is the official language, but many Italians speak other languages, including English.

- Over 98% of people can read and write in their native language.
- Handshakes are an acceptable form of greeting. Closer friends and relations may kiss on the cheek.
- Personal space is often very close, and physical contact such as hugging is acceptable.
- People prefer direct eye contact when communicating.
- It is common to be very emotionally expressive and animated when communicating.

NUTRITION
- Traditional foods include breads, pastas, tomatoes and tomato sauces, vegetables, fruit, cheese, fish, and espresso or strong coffee.
- Red meat is not a common part of the diet.
- Foods are often very rich, with cream sauces and full-fat ice cream, but portions are usually small.
- People of Mediterranean ancestry may be lactose-intolerant.
- Many people drink wine as a regular part of their meals.
- Beer is very common in Italy as well as a traditional lemon liquor called *limoncello.*
- In Italy many people clean out their bodies by drinking bitter greens boiled in water.
- Fast food is becoming more common in this country.
- People may feel offended if an offer for a meal or snack is not accepted.
- "Breaking bread" is an important social custom that signifies friendship and union.
- Italian adults have lower rates of obesity than adults in other European countries, but Italian children have higher rates of obesity than those in other European countries.

PHYSICAL ILLNESS
- Cardiovascular disease is the leading cause of death in Italy.
- Cancers of the respiratory tract, including trachea, bronchus, and lung, are other major causes of death in Italy.

- Colon, rectal, and breast cancer are three other common types in this population.
- Chronic obstructive pulmonary disease, diabetes, and lower respiratory tract infections are other leading causes of death in this country. These diseases are all linked to smoking rates.
- Approximately 22% of Italians are daily smokers.
- Alzheimer's disease and dementia are common causes of death in Italy and occur more often in men.
- Peptic ulcers are routine in this population, which is believed to result from high rates of coffee and alcohol consumption and smoking.
- Health maintenance and preventive medicine, such as health screenings, have gained awareness in recent years.
- In 2005, just under 10% of the Italian population was classified as obese; 48% of men and 34% of women were overweight.
- People may treat a cold by inhaling very hot water and turpentine.

MENTAL ILLNESS

- Mental health issues are generally not considered shameful or stigmatizing, but mental illnesses often go undiagnosed in this country.
- People may believe that their family will help them recover from symptoms of mental illness.
- It is common to be expressive about stress, anger, and happiness.
- Some research suggests that men are more prone to developing symptoms of depression.
- An estimated 5% of Italians younger than 35 years in some urban areas are regular cocaine users.
- Alcoholism is increasing in younger generations, and it has been estimated that around 10% of people younger than 30 years have problems with alcohol.
- Mental health treatment in this country is primarily focused on treating severe conditions, such as schizophrenia and bipolar disorder.

PAIN
- People may be very expressive and vocal about their pain.
- The use of pain medications is widely accepted.

SEXUALITY
- Marriages often last a lifetime in this country, with a divorce rate of 12%, the lowest rate in Europe
- Some Catholics do not believe in the use of birth control.
- Abortion is legal in Italy; however, it is controversial, and rates are low.
- Premarital sex is common, but young men and women often do not become sexually active until their late teens.
- Unmarried cohabitation is very uncommon.
- Babies being born out of wedlock are uncommon in Italy.
- Despite strong religious influences, attitudes about homosexuality are fairly tolerant.
- Teenage pregnancy rates across Italy are low (less than 5%), although the rate is higher (around 10%) in Southern Italy.

CHILDBEARING
- Most women in Italy receive very thorough prenatal care, including genetic counseling, multiple ultrasounds, and regular examinations.
- The father often accompanies the mother during the birth.
- The national birth rate in Italy is 1.26 babies born to each woman on average, which is very low.
- Most mothers stay in the hospital for 3 days after a baby is born in this country, and longer if there are complications.
- In Italy, about 85% of mothers breastfeed initially and about 19% are still breastfeeding at 4–5 months.
- Some people believe the mother should not have sex while she is pregnant.

CHILD REARING

- The average child in Italy attends school for 16 years.
- It is commonly thought that children should be placed in their own beds and rooms at birth and taught to sleep through the night.
- Circumcision is not a common practice.
- Parents may spank their children, although this is becoming less common.
- Sons may be given many more freedoms than daughters.
- In Italy a free education is provided only until age 15, but many people continue their education beyond this point.
- Children are taught to value faith, family, and success.

FAMILY ROLE

- Families are usually very close, and adult children often maintain close relationships with their parents or may live at home into adulthood.
- The father may be emotionally distant from the family but may make many important family decisions.
- The mother may be very close to her children (especially sons) even into adulthood and may have conflicts with them or their spouses when they go against her wishes.
- In this country elders are generally treated with great respect and are cared for at home in their old age.

SPIRITUALITY AND BELIEFS

- 90% of Italians are Catholic; 10% are primarily Protestant or Jewish.
- A Muslim immigrant population is growing in this country and comprised about 2% of the population in 2009.
- Relatively few people attend church regularly in Italy, yet the church exerts a great deal of influence.
- Some people believe that, if they love their family; eat garlic, fresh fruits, and vegetables; and drink a glass of red wine daily, they will not become ill. As such, they may not be receptive to other health maintenance practices.

- Some people in Italy believe that *malocchio* (the evil eye) can make others ill or cause bad things to happen and that drinking cod liver oil will prevent the evil eye.

DEATH AND DYING
- Catholics generally wish to have a priest present near the time of death to provide viaticum (last rites).
- Families may be very vocal and expressive in their grieving, and deaths are often attended by large numbers of family and friends.
- Organ donation and autopsy are sometimes practiced.
- Cremation is not a common practice.
- Living wills and do-not-resuscitate orders are sometimes used in Italy (and may be called "biological will").
- An open-casket viewing at home is traditional.

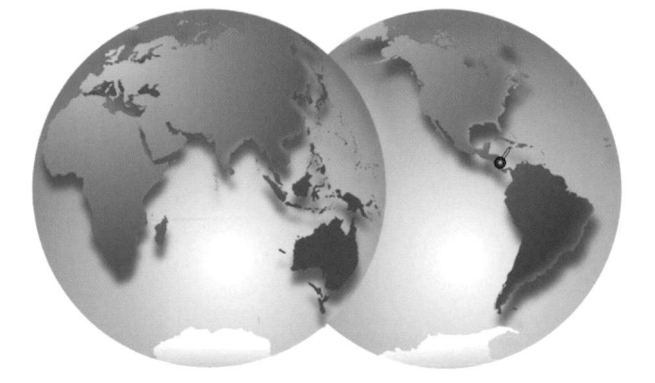

Jamaica

Jamaica is an island nation in the Caribbean Sea, south of the island Cuba. Jamaica is roughly 4500 square miles in size. The population is estimated at about 2.8 million people. Kingston is the largest city and is the nation's capital. The country was originally inhabited by an indigenous population from South America. In 1494, Christopher Columbus landed on the island and claimed it for Spain. The Spanish developed the island to grow sugar and began importing large numbers of slaves from Africa. Jamaica was then captured by the British in 1655, which held the country until 1962, when it became an independent nation. Jamaica has become a mix of people and traditions from many places around the world.

COMMUNICATION
■ The national language is English, but many people speak an English-African Creole.

- Approximately 88% of people can read and write in their native language.
- Eye contact is common, especially during conversations.
- Men may shake hands with direct eye contact. Occasionally, they may lightly tap closed fists in a casual greeting.
- Women greet one another with many handshakes and much hugging.
- Men and women often greet one another with a handshake.
- Personal space is usually about an arm's length.
- People may speak quietly, along with a lot of laughter and animation.
- Communication tends to be direct and honest, and developing harmony is important.

NUTRITION

- Traditional foods include fresh fruits and vegetables, such as plantains, coconuts, and avocados; seafood, and spicy meats, especially chicken.
- People generally prefer to eat natural, unprocessed foods; however, these foods are often fried or cooked in high-fat and high-calorie sauces.
- Tea is a favorite beverage.
- A fruit called *ackee* is popular; if not prepared properly, it can cause the blood sugar to decrease.
- Certain hot and cold foods and beverages are used to treat certain illnesses, which are believed to have hot and cold properties.
- About 54% of adults in Jamaica are overweight, and 24% are obese, with more women than men in these two categories.
- 17% of children 3 and 4 years old are overweight.
- In 2005, about 4% of Jamaican children were considered underweight.
- Iron-deficiency anemia is the primary diet-related problem in Jamaica, with children, teenagers, and pregnant women experiencing it at high rates.
- Jamaican rum is a common alcoholic beverage served in this country at social events.

■ Fast food is popular in Jamaica, with many fast food chains in the country, as well as local-style food chains, which serve jerk foods and other Jamaican favorites.

PHYSICAL ILLNESS

■ Cardiovascular disease, cancer, and diabetes are common causes of death in this country. These result from Jamaica's high rates of obesity.

■ Lower respiratory infections are a major cause of death in Jamaica, with pneumonia and influenza being common health problems.

■ Jamaica has had outbreaks of dengue fever and typhoid fever in recent years.

■ HIV and AIDS are problems, with a rate of 1.2% or about double that of the United States.

■ More young women than men are infected with HIV and die of AIDS in Jamaica. HIV affects about 10% of prostitutes and 30% of homosexual men.

■ Approximately 1 in 300 people has sickle cell anemia.

■ People believe that if a medication does not have physically detectable benefits within a couple of days, then it is not working.

■ Homeopathic remedies are generally thought to be more effective than Western medicine in this culture.

■ If an illness has a sudden onset or is severe, patients often pursue Western medicine remedies; if not, they will likely use naturopathic healers or see a spiritual healer.

■ Illnesses are believed to be caused by either natural influences (such as germs or diet) or by spiritual forces, such as witchcraft or *obeah* (folk magic).

MENTAL ILLNESS

■ Mental illnesses are often considered the result of spiritual influences and must be treated by spiritual healers through the use of herbs, tonics, prayers, and rituals.

- Mentally ill patients who behave violently have been imprisoned in recent years because of a lack of proper treatment facilities.
- Schizophrenia is the most common mental health diagnosis in Jamaica.
- Smoking marijuana is a common practice and is on the rise. In recent years, cocaine, heroin, and ecstasy abuse rates have also increased, partly due to Jamaica being a stopping point for many drugs on their way from Central to North America.
- About 50% of people are regular drinkers, but only about 6% of people surveyed were considered to be problem drinkers.
- Violence and crime are major problems on the island and are thought to be the result of drug and alcohol abuse.
- Rates of homicide and accidental death among young males have risen in the last decade.
- Most mental health treatment available is directed at serious disorders and is not designed to treat depression and anxiety issues.

PAIN
- People are often very expressive about their pain.
- Pain medications are generally considered acceptable.
- Jamaican dogwood and marijuana are sometimes used as traditional pain remedies.

SEXUALITY
- Marriages are not necessarily considered to mean monogamy for men; men frequently have children with more than one woman.
- About 16% of women of childbearing age are married.
- Couples may live together, often with the mother's children by her current partner and from previous relationships as well. Men may come and go between this and other homes.
- It is believed that a woman should attend to her husband's requirements as well as provide many children.

- Homosexuality is considered taboo and illegal. Legislation in Jamaica focuses on homosexual males and states that, if convicted, a man can face up to 10 years in prison. Gangs beat and kill homosexuals or drive them from their homes.
- The rate of teenage pregnancy is very high, with 25% of births in Jamaica being to teenage mothers. This is thought to be due to denial about the risk of getting pregnant, lack of education, and social and cultural misinformation.
- In some poor neighborhoods, women who have not had a child by age 20 years are sometimes called "mules" and are taunted for being "sterile."
- Jamaica has a tradition of "sugar daddies," in which young girls have sex with older men for material gifts.
- Abortion is illegal in Jamaica, including instances when the mother's life is in danger; however, the government estimates that 20,000 to 30,000 illegal abortions are performed annually in the country.
- Some women believe that douching with Pepsi after intercourse or having intercourse in the ocean will prevent pregnancy.

CHILDBEARING
- In Jamaica, 53% of pregnant women were found to be anemic, along with 34% of lactating women.
- Many birthing facilities test for sickle cell anemia shortly after birth.
- Women with sickle cell anemia have higher rates of miscarriage, still-birth, and perinatal mortality.
- About 22% of women still breastfeed at 6 months.
- A birth is considered private, and only trained birthing attendants are present during a delivery. People believe that too many outsiders can spread infections and put spells on the baby.
- Asafetida, an herb, is placed on the newborn for its protection, and a bible is often kept open on or near the bed.
- A piece of red cloth may be tied around the baby's wrist to give the baby strength.

- Most pregnancies, from prenatal care to labor and delivery, are handled by a midwife.
- Thyme tea is often given to women after a birth as it is believed to have effects similar to oxytocin, which helps to contract the uterus.

CHILD REARING
- Children attend school for an average of 12 years in this country.
- Baby formula is considered a status symbol, but the formula is sometimes not diluted properly (to save money), which results in malnutrition for the infant.
- Approximately 4% of children in Jamaica are malnourished. This results in children who are stunted and have cognitive impairments.
- Approximately 1 in 250 children born in Jamaica has sickle cell anemia, which is often most serious in children. Infants have a morbidity rate from 5% to 13% by 2 years of age, depending on the severity of the disease.
- Physical punishment has been banned by the Jamaican government, but it is still a common practice among some parents.
- Jamaican schools report higher levels of attention deficit, adjustment, and conduct disorders, which some believe is the result of watching too much television and poor parental supervision.
- Children are raised to be seen and not heard in many Jamaican households.

FAMILY ROLE
- The family unit often consists of a grandmother, a mother, and her children (often by different fathers). The fathers may be involved, be absent, or come and go from the family. Often, children from another family member, such as an aunt or cousin, are included in the family unit.
- The adult female will often make the decisions for her family unit.

- The family often provides much of a sick patient's care and brings all meals from home.
- Jamaica is considered a male-dominated society, but more than half of all households are headed by women.
- Women are generally considered to be in charge in times of illness.

SPIRITUALITY AND BELIEFS
- The majority of people in Jamaica are Christians, with influences from other religions, such as Baha'i and Islam.
- Christianity is more common in affluent families; rural and low-income families are more likely to practice voodoo.
- Rastafarian is a religious movement that incorporates African and Jamaican culture with Christianity; it rejects Western society.
- Animal sacrifices are sometimes made to promote healing.
- Western medicine is often pursued only when traditional healers have failed.
- When a child has asthma, one traditional cure entails placing the child under a banana tree and then chopping the tree down.

DEATH AND DYING
- The family will weep and cry loudly at the time of death of a loved one.
- After death the family may be very concerned that the deceased will turn into a ghost. Ghosts are widely feared in this culture.
- The family may wish to wash and wrap the body in preparation for the funeral.
- A body must be carried out feet first due to cultural and religious beliefs.
- A celebratory wake may take place to appease the ghost and make it harmless.
- Autopsies are permitted, but organ donation is not generally performed.

- The deceased may be buried with a knife to protect the person from witchcraft or a cell phone for communication.
- Funerals are often large and emotional gatherings that reflect on the status and wealth of the deceased and the family.
- Cremation is very uncommon.

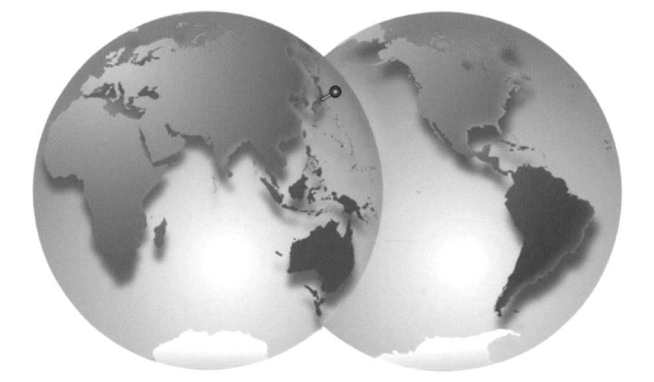

Japan

Japan is a country in the Pacific Ocean composed of over 3000 islands, although four main islands account for 97% of the country's land mass. With more than 128 million inhabitants, Japan is the 10th most populous country, but it ranks only 61st in terms of size. Much of the land that composes Japan is uninhabitable, and as a result the country has some of the most densely populated regions in the world.

Japan is a constitutional monarchy, with the emperor having limited power and serving mostly as a symbolic representation of the country and its history. The deciding government officials are the prime minister and the other elected representatives. Japan has the third largest economy in the world, with finance, high technology, motor vehicles, and real estate being the major industries. Most Japanese people enjoy an elevated standard of living, good salaries, and excellent education in this highly developed country.

COMMUNICATION

- The national language is Japanese.
- 99% of people can read and write in their native language.
- People generally have great respect for their elders and authority figures.
- The most common and acceptable greeting in Japan is to bow with the hands at the sides, although this is not expected from a non-Japanese person.
- Handshakes are becoming more common; patting another person on the back or head (especially an elderly person) may be considered disrespectful.
- Entering a room and introducing oneself to the elderly persons first demonstrates respect.
- Some people may offer limited eye contact, especially when speaking with a person considered authoritative.
- Smiling can indicate a range of emotions, including anger, happiness, nervousness, or discomfort.
- Nodding does not always indicate agreement.
- People may not ask questions, even when they are unsure.
- Particularly in older generations, shame may be a powerful emotion, and maintaining self-respect may be considered important.
- It may be considered rude to refuse a gift if one is offered. It is appropriate to receive a gift with both hands and to open it later away from the giver.

NUTRITION

- The traditional diet consists of rice, vegetables, fruit, noodles, tofu, and seafood.
- The traditional diet is generally very healthy; however, it can be high in sodium. This is primarily due to the sauces in which many are foods cooked and to the smoked fish in the diet.
- Green or Chinese teas are a very important remedy in Japan.

- Ginger, sake, and eggs are believed to promote recovery when ingested during a cold.
- Meals often consist of several courses, each course consisting of relatively small portions.
- In Japan, 24% of people older than 15 years are considered overweight and 5% obese, which is lower than most developed countries. Nevertheless, these rates are on the rise.

PHYSICAL ILLNESS

- Preventive health care is valued, through diet, exercise, and health screenings.
- Hygiene is very important.
- The leading causes of death in Japan are cardiovascular disease, followed by lower respiratory infections.
- Cancer is the third major cause of death in this country, with trachea, bronchus, and lung cancers being the most common. Following are stomach, colon, liver and rectal cancers.
- Japan has very high rates of smoking relative to other developed countries, which is linked to increased rates of cancer and respiratory infections.
- In Japan 43% of adult males and 13% of adult females smoke.
- Japanese Americans have a higher rate of diabetes type II than Caucasian Americans. In the past decade diabetes type II has been on the rise in Japan.
- There have been outbreaks of severe acute respiratory syndrome in Japan in recent years.

MENTAL ILLNESS

- Particularly for older generations, shame may be a powerful force. Shaming oneself or one's family may be emotionally devastating.
- Mental illness has carried a social stigma, and the family of a patient may not want the patient to receive mental health treatment. Attitudes are changing, however, particularly among younger generations.

- Therapy is not generally well received, and mental health treatment is limited. In Japan, there are only two mental health hospitals, with 200 beds each.
- Particularly in the past, mental illness was considered caused by an individual's own bad behavior.
- Suicide is a major problem in Japan and is the leading cause of death for people younger than 30 years, although it is also common in other age groups. Approximately three-fourths of Japanese suicides annually are male.
- In the past, Japan's military culture had a tradition of honorable suicide (for example, *kamikaze*), and this has influenced what some call a "tolerant" attitude toward suicide in Japan. Government efforts are being made to counteract this and lower national suicide rates.
- Dementia is common, in part because of long life expectancy (although it is not clear what other factors may also be relevant). In Japan, dementia is often underdiagnosed and undertreated.
- In some cases, patients may vocalize the physical symptoms underlying psychological issues. For example, a patient may detail stress-related stomach pains instead of saying she is feeling very stressed.
- It is estimated that alcoholism afflicts 2% of the Japanese population, and 50% of men report drinking on a regular basis.
- Japan has limited treatment programs for alcoholism.
- Drug abuse rates are generally lower than those of other developed countries; however, rates relating to cannabis and ecstasy are rising.
- Child abuse is a concern in Japan: nearly 47,000 cases of child abuse were reported in 2008, and this number is increasing.

PAIN

- People often believe they should tolerate pain and not express their discomfort.
- People may refuse pain medications.

■ Patients may have higher pain tolerances than patients from other countries.

■ Rectal pain medications are more likely to be refused . Oral medications are generally preferred.

SEXUALITY

■ Female patients of older generations may dress and act modestly, as this is a traditional value. Younger generations are likely to behave and dress far more casually.

■ The most common form of birth control in this country is the condom, which, along with low rates of intravenous drug use, may have contributed to low rates of HIV.

■ Homosexuality is not illegal in Japan; however, there is some discrimination against homosexuals.

■ About a third of Japanese women have been victims of domestic abuse.

■ Japan has the lowest teenage birth rate in the industrialized world, with only 4 out of every 1000 teenage girls giving birth.

■ Babies born out of wedlock are relatively uncommon and have traditionally carried some social stigma.

■ Abortion is not discussed openly but is legal in this country.

CHILDBEARING

■ The average woman in Japan has 1.21 children.

■ Boys have traditionally been preferred, although female children have become more valued; in some cases this may be because females are thought to more likely care for their parents into old age.

■ Prenatal care is generally accepted.

■ Vaginal delivery is frequently preferred.

■ Fathers may not think it is appropriate to be in the delivery room.

■ Breastfeeding and bottle feeding at the same time is common in Japan, and infants are usually breastfed for 3–4 months.

CHILD REARING

- The average child in Japan attends school for 15–16 years, and many go on to attend university.
- Education is very competitive in Japan and can be very stressful for children.
- Male circumcision is common in Japan.
- Children are taught to be polite, quiet, and humble.
- Parents are often permissive with young children.

FAMILY ROLE

- The male is usually the head of the family.
- Success at work is likely to be a major priority in a Japanese man's life. A person's profession is a very important part of one's life and identity.
- In the past a close family network was an important part of Japanese life; this may now be less significant for some families.
- The family may prefer to provide physical care for a patient.
- Individuals may be considered less important than the family unit.
- Many single mothers in Japan are poor and are forced to work, often in the sex industry, in order support themselves and their children.
- With the help of their adult children, elderly family members are generally cared for in their homes as long as possible. The number of people in retirement homes has also increased significantly in recent decades.

SPIRITUALITY AND BELIEFS

- Buddhism and Shintoism are the main religions in Japan and together (often as a synthesis of the two religions) are the religions of most people. Christians make up about 2% of the population.
- People may adhere to and perform rituals from more than one religion (e.g., Buddhist, Shinto, Christian).
- Although many Japanese are affiliated with temples and engage in various religious rituals, many others are agnostic.

- Buddhists believe that people must be in harmony with themselves, the universe, and society in order to have good health.
- Conformity in the Japanese culture used to be an important value, but individualism is beginning to have an influence.

DEATH AND DYING

- Some family members may feel very strongly about not telling a terminally ill patient about the prognosis; however, in a recent Japanese study, 65% of people surveyed stated they would want full disclosure if they had a terminal diagnosis.
- People sometimes commit suicide after learning they have a terminal illness.
- In Japan, autopsies are performed when the cause of death is questionable.
- Organ donation is not generally accepted.
- It is often considered very important that the body of the deceased be clean and the orifices be blocked with cotton or gauze.
- Japan passed legislation in 1995 legalizing assisted suicide for those with severe pain and an impending death; however, this practice has not been implemented widely.
- Nearly all people are cremated.
- The average cost of a funeral in Japan is more expensive than in any other country.
- Most people in Japan practice Buddhist rituals after death. This includes wetting the deceased's lips with water and placing flowers, incense, and a candle on a small table near the body. A knife may also be placed on the chest of the body to drive away "evil spirits."
- The family may wish to position the body so the head is facing north or west, representing the realm of the Buddha.

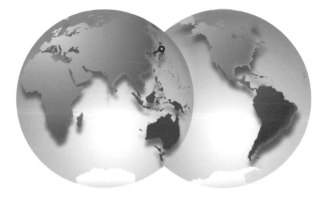

Korea

Korea is a country united on the Korean Peninsula just south of China. Korea has a long history, with human fossils having been found in the region dating back over 100,000 years and ancient pottery remains dating back over 10,000 years. In 1948, the country was divided by war. The United States backed the pro-democracy faction, and Russia backed the pro-communist faction. This eventually led to the country splitting along the 38th parallel into two separate nations. Many Koreans believe that they are still one people.

Today South Korea, or the Republic of Korea, is a democracy with more than 50 million people. South Korea occupies about 38,600 square miles, making it the third most populated country in the world. Seoul is the capitol of South Korea and the second largest metropolitan city in the world.

North Korea, or the Democratic People's Republic of Korea, is a communist country located on the northern part of the Korean peninsula. North Korea is ruled by the dictator Kim Jong-Il and is considered by many to be a totalitarian Stalinist government. North Koreans are completely unable to communicate with anyone outside the country, including South Koreans, and have very limited access to health care and, some say, even food. There are around 24 million people living on 46,500 square miles. North Korea is of great interest to the international community due to concerns about human rights and the country's recent development as a nuclear threat to South Korea and the world with its attempts to build a missile.

COMMUNICATION

- The primary language of North and South Korea is Korean.
- In North Korea a reported 99% of people can read and write Korean. In South Korea an estimated 98% of people can read and write in their native language.
- It is traditional to greet people by their proper title and with a small bow, especially if the person being greeted is an elder.
- Proper titles, such as Mrs., Miss., Ms., or Mr., are appreciated.
- Interpreters are generally appreciated when trying to communicate with non-Korean speakers.
- Physical contact is not generally acceptable, unless it is part of a physical examination or medical care.
- Direct eye contact is not common during communication.
- Silence is a major part of communication.
- When giving an item to another person, it is best to use both hands as this shows respect and the value of the item being given.
- Some people believe they must give the nurse or care provider a gift or money in order to receive good care.
- Standing with two hands behind the back is considered rude in this culture, as is allowing the sole of the foot to face in the direction of another person.

NUTRITION

- Traditional foods include rice, vegetables, meat, and fruit.
- The sodium content of traditional Korean foods is often high.
- Malnutrition is a major problem in North Korea, as food is scarce.
- Many people are lactose-intolerant and avoid dairy products.
- Conditions are believed to have hot and cold qualities, which are not related to temperature. To restore balance in the body, certain foods and drinks may be necessary. For example, kidney disease is a "hot condition" and requires treatment with "cold" foods, which may be served warm.

PHYSICAL ILLNESS

- Major causes of death in South Korea include cardiovascular disease, diabetes, cirrhosis of the liver, accidents, and injuries.
- In North Korea, major causes of death include cardiovascular disease, lower respiratory infections, perinatal conditions, chronic obstructive pulmonary disease, diabetes, stomach cancer, violence, and famine.
- The most common types of cancer in South Korea include tracheal, bronchial, lung, stomach, and liver.
- North Korea has had major outbreaks of severe acute respiratory syndrome in recent years, as well as typhoid and cholera.
- Rates of tuberculosis infections are high in North and South Korea.
- North and South Korea have high rates of hepatitis infections and malaria.
- People are often very sensitive to feelings of cold.
- Air and water pollution are major problems in North Korea.
- Vomiting is considered embarrassing, and people are often hesitant to discuss it.
- Bowel issues are also very embarrassing and not readily discussed.
- Use of oxygen is believed to indicate that the patient's condition is very serious or life-threatening.
- Acupressure and massage are believed to be very beneficial for health promotion.

MENTAL ILLNESS
- Mental illnesses carry a great social stigma, and patients may refuse treatment or medications to avoid being stigmatized.
- Suicide rates are on the rise in South Korea.
- The rates of reported mental illnesses are increasing in South Korea; major diagnoses are dementia and delayed mental development as well as mood disorders such as depression.
- In North Korea, people are sometimes diagnosed as having "anger syndrome," which is the inability to cope with stress.

PAIN
- Patients, especially men, may not openly express their pain.
- Pain medication is generally accepted.

SEXUALITY
- Some female patients may prefer same-sex providers for reproductive issues.
- Modesty is often very important for Korean patients, who want to remain covered as much as possible.
- In North Korea people of the same sex may hold hands as friends only.
- Expressions of love and affection are often very subtle.
- In North Korea, public displays of affection are considered unacceptable.
- Homosexuality in South Korea is not generally accepted, and the legal system does not provide the same protections for homosexuals as it does for straight people.
- Homosexuality in North Korea is not often discussed, but it is generally believed that homosexuals are at most tolerated.

CHILDBEARING
- Specific food choices during pregnancy are believed to influence the intelligence, beauty, and personality of the baby.
- Dairy products are not a common part of the Korean diet, which may cause expectant mothers to be low in calcium.

- At the time of birth until 7 weeks post partum, the mother must eat only warm foods.
- The father is commonly in the delivery room at the time of birth.
- Mothers often do not have strong feelings regarding vaginal deliveries or cesarean sections.
- Expectant mothers may be very vocal during deliveries, while older family members are sometimes embarrassed by this and may try to quiet them.
- It is often best to inform the father first of any problems with the infant. Mothers commonly blame themselves for any problems.
- Male children are sometimes circumcised.

CHILD REARING
- Male children are generally preferred.
- In North Korea children may occasionally not wear clothing.
- Sometimes children are not encouraged to become independent but are instead encouraged not to challenge their place in society.
- In South Korea, education is considered a child's first priority.
- Mothers often are more permissive, and fathers are the disciplinarians.

FAMILY ROLE
- Children may be expected to provide physical care to the elder family members.
- A person's self-esteem is often directly tied to identification with the family.
- Families are generally hierarchal, with males having slightly more status and decision-making opportunities than female members.
- A family member will often stay in the hospital with the patient and help to provide care.
- Elders are generally cared for at home, and nursing homes are considered a last resort.

SPIRITUALITY AND BELIEFS

■ North Korea is traditionally Buddhist and Confucian, with some Christians. The North Korean government closely regulates all religious activities, and many religious practices are forbidden.

■ About 50% of South Koreans do not claim a religious affiliation; about 26% are Christian (19% Protestant and 6% Catholic); and 24% are Buddhist.

■ Many people are fatalistic and believe that luck or something they did may have caused their illness.

■ Shamans may be used to remove an "evil spirit" from a patient or to promote spiritual healing.

DEATH AND DYING

■ Visitors may chant or burn incense near a dying patient.

■ Family members may want to wash the body of the deceased.

■ Family members often prefer to be told first about a bad diagnosis so they may tell the ill patient or choose not to tell.

■ Organ donation and autopsy are not commonly accepted.

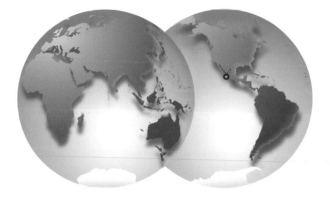

Mexico

Mexico is located on the southernmost portion of North America. It is the 14th largest country and the 11th most populous, with about 111 million people. Mexico City is the 10th largest city and is built on the ruins of the ancient Aztec city of Tenochtitlán. Many Mexicans are descendants of the Aztecs and the Spanish who conquered them. Almost 90% of Mexicans are Catholic, although Mexico has no official religion. Recent battles between drug cartels and the government have greatly jeopardized the stability of this developing country.

COMMUNICATION
■ The national language is Spanish.
■ 91% of the people can read and write in their native language.
■ Handshakes are a common and acceptable greeting.

■ When being addressed, Mexicans appreciate proper titles.
■ Men are considered the head of the family and are generally addressed first.
■ The head of the family may speak on behalf of other family members.
■ Standing with the hands on hips is considered a confrontational stance.
■ To avoid confrontation, people may avoid saying "no" and may say "yes" or "we'll see."
■ It is considered unacceptable for a woman to discuss reproductive issues in front of a man.
■ People may be uncomfortable being asked direct questions regarding their immigration or marital status.

NUTRITION
■ The traditional diet consists primarily of corn, rice, beans, and vegetables.
■ Many people have diets that are high in sodium and fat from fried foods and added salt.
■ Illnesses are believed to have hot and cold qualities, which are not necessarily related to temperature. To restore balance in the body, certain foods and drinks may be necessary. For example, kidney disease is a "hot condition" and requires treatment with "cold" foods, which may actually be served warm. Dairy products and tomatoes are considered cold foods, and alcohol and onions are hot foods.
■ Mexicans may prefer beverages without ice.
■ Being overweight may be viewed as healthy.
■ Many people are Catholic and avoid eating meat on Fridays.

PHYSICAL ILLNESS
■ People may believe that the use of oxygen indicates that the patient's condition is very serious or life-threatening.
■ Diabetes is a major cause of death in Mexico and is often undiagnosed.

- Cardiovascular disease is another leading cause of death in Mexico.
- Cervical cancer is common.
- Accidents and homicides comprise about 12% of deaths in Mexico and are often drug- and alcohol-related.
- Smoking is a common practice in Mexico and contributes to many health problems, such as high rates of chronic obstructive pulmonary disease, perinatal complications, and lower respiratory tract infections.
- Mexico City has the world's most polluted air.
- Cirrhosis is a major cause of death in Mexico because of high rates of alcoholism and hepatitis.
- Mexico has the second highest rate of obesity, second only to the United States, with obesity affecting about 70% of the population.
- Self-care is generally not considered beneficial in this culture, and ambulation may not be well received. Many people believe it is important for the patient to rest.
- Patients may not understand what a prescription is and may expect the health-care provider to give them the medication, as is the practice in Mexico.
- Herbal teas are often an important remedy.
- Some people believe that covering a patient with many blankets will make them "sweat out" a fever.
- "Cupping" involves placing a heated glass bowl over a body part to relieve discomfort.
- Some herbal supplements from Mexico, such as arzarcon or greta, may contain lead and mercury.
- A raw egg is sometimes placed on the body to dispel the "evil eye," which is often believed to cause physical symptoms.

MENTAL ILLNESS

- The words "mental illness" and "counseling" carry a stigma and bring shame on the person and the family.

- Depression is considered shameful and frequently goes untreated.
- Psychotherapy is used to treat only severe mental illnesses in Mexico.
- *Susto* means "fright" and can be displayed by panic, nervousness, despondency, anorexia, or diarrhea. It is believed to be caused by bad news or events.
- Domestic violence is a major problem in Mexico and is usually ignored.
- In 2009, the Mexican government legalized small quantities of heroin, cocaine, marijuana, and amphetamines. Nevertheless, drug abuse is less common in Mexico than in the United States.
- Alcoholism rates are highest among men who have emigrated to the United States from Mexico.

PAIN
- Patients are often stoic and do not express pain.
- Men frequently do not communicate pain or their need for pain medication.

SEXUALITY
- People generally prefer same-sex care providers and believe that only male providers and spouses should touch a male patient's genitals.
- Modesty is important, and it is best to keep the patient covered as much as possible.
- Homosexuality is generally not tolerated; there is some violence against homosexuals.
- Women may be extremely secretive about the use of birth control due to cultural and religious beliefs.
- Abortion is illegal in some parts of Mexico, so women obtain abortions from clinics and "back alley" providers.
- The rhythm method is commonly practiced in Mexico.

- Pregnancy during adolescence is very common in Mexico, and to some it is a sign of becoming an adult or reaching maturity.
- Extramarital affairs, generally by husbands only, are accepted in some groups.

CHILDBEARING

- About one in four pregnant women from Mexico is anemic.
- Male children are generally preferred.
- Pica, which is the craving to consume non-nutritive substances, is common among pregnant women.
- People may believe that a pregnant woman should not raise her arms over her head because doing so will loop the umbilical cord around the baby's neck.
- Some people believe that unsatisfied cravings of the pregnant woman will cause harm to the baby.
- Women often observe a lying-in period after a baby is born. This period lasts approximately 6 weeks and is a time during which the mother rests, stays very warm, and avoids bathing.
- In parts of Mexico, herbal tea is believed to encourage contractions.
- Women believe that colostrum is unhealthy and do not breastfeed until their milk comes in.
- It is commonly thought that a mother's milk is inadequate and must be supplemented with formula.
- Breastfeeding is not common in this country. Women are often uncomfortable exposing their breasts, and men from Mexico often disapprove of nursing.
- Mothers may believe that air can enter the baby through the umbilicus, so they may wrap a band around the abdomen until the cord falls off.

CHILD REARING

■ Children generally attend school for an average of 13 years in Mexico.

■ Elders are more revered than children.

■ A depressed fontanel is treated by pressing on the soft palate and holding the baby upside down over a dish of water or applying a soap mash to the fontanel.

■ Many people believe that a curse, or "evil eye," can result from an infant being praised too much. Too much praise can cause others to be envious of the child and thereby lead to a curse.

■ Hispanic infants may have mongolian spots, which are dark discolorations on the skin that resemble bruises.

■ Children are often expected to work at a young age.

■ Anemia is very common in children from Mexico.

FAMILY ROLE

■ In a traditional Mexican family, males are the head of the family and often make decisions on behalf of all family members.

■ Male migrant workers may have more than one family.

■ The needs of the family take precedence over the needs of any individual member.

■ Family members often take care of sick members.

SPIRITUALITY AND BELIEFS

■ Most people in Mexico are Roman Catholic.

■ Some people believe that a person's health is out of his or her control and is only in the hands of God.

■ Some people believe only a priest can remove the "curse" that is causing a person to be ill.

■ Compliments unaccompanied by a friendly touch are sometimes believed to cause an "evil eye."

DEATH AND DYING

■ People of the Catholic faith generally wish to have a priest present near the time of death to provide viaticum, or last rites.

■ Children are not exposed to the concepts of death or dying.

■ It is very important that a person not die alone.

■ Family members often want to remain with a body to ensure it is treated properly.

■ In Mexico new legislation is increasing awareness about do not resuscitate orders and the refusal of treatment for terminally ill patients.

■ Organ donations and transplants have become a more established practice in Mexico in recent years.

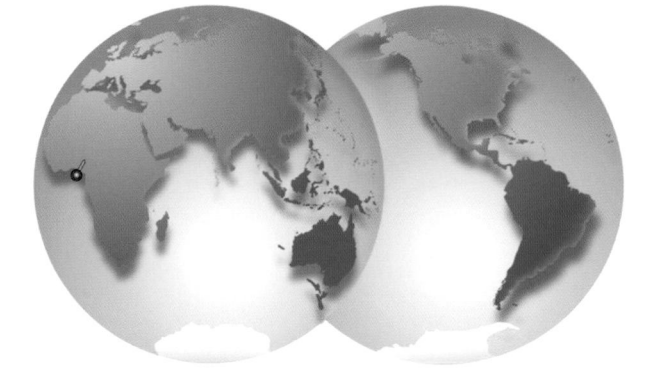

Nigeria

The Federal Republic of Nigeria is a country in Western Africa. This country is the eighth most populated country in the world and the most populated country on the African continent. There are 149 million people, and the population is growing very quickly. Nigeria covers slightly less than 357,000 square miles, making it the world's 32nd largest country. Archaeological data record people in the region from 9000 B.C. During colonial times, Nigeria became a British colony. After World War II, the country gained its independence and became Nigeria, named after the Niger River, which flows through the country. In the past few decades, this country has seen political instability after a number of military coups. In 1999, the population elected a new president and established a democracy; however, there have been extensive claims of election fraud. In recent years, efforts have been made to reduce government corruption. Nigeria has large amounts of petroleum, making it one of the fastest-growing economies.

COMMUNICATION
- The national language is English, but there are more than 10 commonly spoken ethnic minority languages.
- Nigeria is roughly divided into North, South, and East, with predominant languages in these regions being Hausa, Yoruba, and Igbo, respectively. Several other minority languages are also common.
- In this country, about 68% of people can read and write their native language.
- People generally greet one another by shaking hands. Followers of Islam, who comprise about 40% of the population, do not shake hands with people of the opposite sex. In these instances, men wait for the woman to extend her hand when greeting.
- A sincere smile is important when greeting and shaking hands.
- A slight bow of the head when greeting an elder is considered respectful.
- Rushing a greeting is considered very rude.
- People generally prefer to be addressed using a proper name with Mr., Miss, or Mrs. or their professional title.
- Close personal space is acceptable.
- Eye contact is somewhat limited as people may look at the person while they speak but look away while the other person answers.
- Faith and natural healers are usually not discussed with providers of Western medicine.
- People may be hesitant to share information with outsiders because they fear being judged or misunderstood.

NUTRITION
- People often do not take in enough essential vitamins and minerals, which may result in malnutrition, abnormal blood characteristics, stunted growth, and a wide variety of health problems.

- Traditional foods are very spicy and flavorful and often include rice, beans, and vegetables.
- Lactose intolerance is common.
- The largest meal of the day is traditionally served in the late afternoon.
- All foods are generally served cooked; even raw vegetables are not common.
- Many people prefer fried foods and foods that are high in sodium.
- Muslims do not eat pork.
- It is believed that eating too many rich foods causes "high blood" and that consuming too few causes "low blood." The cure for high blood is to eat white-colored foods, and the cure for low blood is to eat red, rich foods.
- Food and mealtimes are very important. Patients may benefit greatly by partaking in family meals when possible.
- Rates of malnutrition are high due to droughts resulting from climate change, poor soil quality, and a high birth rate of 7.1 children per woman, making food very scarce.
- Alcohol is commonly served at meals and social events, except in Muslim communities. Beer is a very popular beverage, and traditional drinks, such as palm wine, are also common.

PHYSICAL ILLNESS
- AIDS is the primary cause of death.
- Lower respiratory tract infections are the second leading cause of death, followed by malaria, diarrheal diseases, and measles.
- Tuberculosis is a major problem and is one of the top ten causes of death.
- Sickle cell anemia is common.
- Hypertension is common, especially for adult males.
- Hepatitis A and E are common, resulting from contact with body fluids and poor sanitation.
- Parasitic infections are common in rural areas.

- People often form keloid scar tissue on surgical sites or where skin trauma has occurred; even minor razor nicks can result in a keloid scar.
- Family members may wrap an ill person in blankets and provide hot drinks so the person can sweat out the illness.
- People may share their medications with other family members, leading to incomplete courses of treatment
- Rates of obesity are on the rise in more affluent regions.
- The life expectancy is just under 50 years.

MENTAL ILLNESS
- Mental illnesses are often thought to be the result of spiritual imbalances in the person who is experiencing symptoms.
- Psychiatric medications are largely unavailable.
- People often refer to depression as feeling tired, but they are frequently open to treatment.
- Alcohol use is common; however, rates of reported health and behavior problems associated with alcoholism are low.
- Drug abuse rates are high especially in men. Commonly abused drugs include cannabis, benzodiazepines, cocaine, heroin, and zakami and paw paw leaves, which are locally grown plants.

PAIN
- People may express pain openly and accept pain medications.
- People frequently attribute pain to being in the rain or cold air.
- Acetaminophen and other pain relievers may cause gastrointestinal discomfort.
- Some research shows that larger doses of pain relievers are required to achieve pain relief.
- Chili pepper powder is sometimes applied as a polstice for pain; it contains capsaicin, which does have pain-relieving properties.

SEXUALITY

- Same-sex providers are generally preferred.
- Men are considered to be the head of households.
- Homosexuality is illegal and is punishable by stoning to death in some states and a minimum of 14 years in prison throughout the country.
- Men may have multiple wives.
- Oral contraceptives are the most common type of birth control.
- Rhythm method is another common form of birth control, usually because other contraceptives are unavailable.
- Female genital mutilation is common, affecting 30%–100% of women, depending on the region of the country.
- It is estimated that up to half of the women have experienced physical, sexual, or psychological abuse within the family.
- Female Muslims may cover their entire bodies and may be very resistant to removing this covering.
- People often become sexually active at a young age and often do not use contraceptives.
- AIDS is the leading cause of death of women between the ages of 25 and 44 years.
- HIV is usually transmitted through heterosexual intercourse.
- Abortion is illegal, except to save the life of the mother; however, illegal abortions are very common and are frequently performed in clinics, sometimes in an unsafe manner.
- Rates of teenage pregnancy are high.

CHILDBEARING

- Perinatal complications comprise a major cause of death, resulting from lack of medical care for pregnant women, especially in rural areas.
- Only 31% of women give birth in health-care facilities.
- About 60% of women have access to prenatal care.
- Female family members are often the only ones in a delivery room.

- Women frequently prefer vaginal deliveries.
- Mothers will generally stay in bed for 40 days after a delivery while family members assist in caring for other children.
- Cold drafts blowing on the mother during the delivery are thought to thicken the maternal blood and cause complications.
- Mothers are often willing to breastfeed if they are educated and encouraged to do so.
- Male children are sometimes circumcised.
- Children are often named on the 8th day of life in a naming ceremony.

CHILD REARING
- The average child attends school for 8 years.
- Infants often have lower birth weights than infants from other countires.
- Parents often believe it is best to introduce solid foods at about 2 months of age.
- The "evil eye" is a curse upon a child that is brought on by someone's evil thoughts or envy of the baby.
- Child discipline is very strict, and children are expected to help their parents.
- Neighbors often participate in raising the children in their community.
- Children are taught to value the family, and female children are taught that they will have a husband and children.
- Nigeria has an estimated 1.8 million orphans due to HIV and AIDS.
- Homeless children sometimes sniff solvents to get high.

FAMILY ROLE
- Fathers often make the final decisions on behalf of all family members.
- Many families are single-parent households, with a mother raising the children.
- Divorce is taboo, but it is possible to obtain a divorce, and divorce rates are increasing.

■ Marriage often unites two families, so a divorce affects many family members.

■ Elders are usually cared for at home, but elder care homes are becoming more common in some urban areas.

■ Families are often decimated due to high rates of HIV and AIDS, with children often having the disease.

SPIRITUALITY AND BELIEFS

■ About 50% of people are Muslim, and about 40% are Christian.

■ People use a mix of Western medicine, voodoo, faith healing, and natural remedies.

■ Nigerians believe that illness is either the result of natural causes and "God's will," or unnatural causes and the "devil's will."

■ People may believe that having enough faith can cure a sick person.

DEATH AND DYING

■ Families may wish to have an older family member communicate a bad diagnosis to the patient.

■ Families may choose to keep an ill relative at home until near death but then moved back to the hospital. Dying at home is considered bad luck.

■ Organ and blood donations are not usually acceptable.

■ The family may grieve loudly and for a long time.

■ People may resist canceling life support or signing do-not-resuscitate (DNR) orders. They may be waiting for a miracle to save the patient.

■ For Muslims it is important never to give up hope, so hospice, DNR orders, and living wills are generally not well received.

■ Elaborate funerals are common and may take weeks to plan while the body is kept in a mortuary.

■ Muslim families may wish to bury the deceased before sun sets on the day the person dies.

■ Many people prefer to be buried in their native country and may purchase enough life insurance to ensure that the body can be flown home after death.

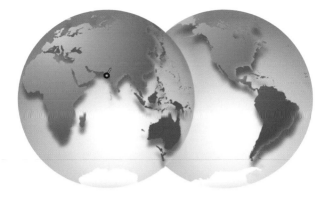

Pakistan

The Islamic Republic of Pakistan is located in South Asia. The country's population is estimated at over 176 million people, which makes Pakistan the sixth most populous country in the world and the second largest Muslim population. Pakistan is also the 36th largest country by area, covering over 340,000 square miles. It is an Islamic republic with an elected prime minister. The Indus Valley is one of the oldest sites of known civilizations and spans most of what is present-day Pakistan.

COMMUNICATION
- The official language is Urdu. Many people also speak English, and there are several regional dialects, such as Punjabi, Pashto, Saraiki, Sindhi, Kashmiri, and Balochi.

- About half the population is unable to read in any language.
- Men generally greet each other with a handshake or a hug, but women do not greet with any kind of physical contact.
- People generally do not use first names .
- Direct eye contact is not common and may make some people uncomfortable.
- People prefer expansive personal space.
- People prefer a soft tone of voice and attitudes of humility, modesty, and tolerance.
- Silence is often appreciated and conveys acceptance.
- Older people may respond with stories rather than address a question or a subject directly.
- Signing consents may cause some people to feel unsure, and they may need additional explanations and reassurances that this is a standard practice.

NUTRITION

- Flavorful wheat flatbread, lentils, and vegetables are common foods.
- Lunch is generally the largest meal.
- Pakistan is making major efforts to improve access to clean water; otherwise, water in Pakistan may contain parasites, arsenic, nitrates, and fluoride.
- Meal times are usually serious; this is time during which people express gratitude for the food being eaten.
- Certain hot and cold foods are thought to promote recovery for certain illnesses.
- Sweet foods are not a common part of the diet.
- Fish, red meat, and certain fruits are considered unhealthy when eaten with dairy products.
- During Ramadan, a religious holiday that lasts for 1 month and occurs on varying dates, people fast each day until sundown.

- Nutritional deficiencies are common, particularly among women; for example, more than 40% of women in Pakistan are anemic.
- In accordance with Islam, alcohol consumption is rare.

PHYSICAL ILLNESS
- Conditions of the respiratory tract are a major cause of death in this country: lower respiratory tract infections comprise the primary cause of death.
- Tuberculosis, chronic obstructive pulmonary disease, and whooping cough are the leading causes of death in Pakistan.
- Cardiovascular disease is also a major cause of death.
- In the past 10 years, two major earthquakes occurred, killing and injuring hundreds of thousands of people and leading to increased rates of disease and malnutrition rates.
- Domestic violence is not explicitly prohibited in Pakistan and therefore may be considered "a private or family matter."
- Abuses such as bride burning, honor killings, and child marriage have become less common in the last decade, but they still occur in more rural populations.
- People do not believe in self-care during illness and are generally very passive regarding their care.
- Nausea and vomiting are thought to be beneficial because they expel poisons and toxins from the body.
- People sometimes do not understand that germs cause illnesses, and therefore they may not wash their hands or clean their wounds to prevent infections.
- Rates of HIV and AIDS infections are very low in this country, involving mainly IV drug users.

MENTAL ILLNESS
- Mental illness carries a great social stigma.
- People often seek medical help only for severe mental illnesses and may describe their concerns as physical symptoms instead.

- Recent studies show anxiety and depression may be as high as 34%.
- Access to psychiatric medications and therapy is limited in this country, especially in rural areas.
- Pakistan is one of the world's largest exporters of heroin, and rates of heroin abuse in the country are increasing.

PAIN

- People may not feel comfortable expressing pain.
- Care providers may need to ask specific questions to determine the nature of a patient's pain.
- Islam forbids the use of narcotics, so narcotic pain relievers may not be accepted.
- Some people believe that pain relievers may not be used on religious holidays.

SEXUALITY

- Talking about sexual organs is generally not acceptable.
- In Pakistan, women often cover their whole bodies and may be very uncomfortable with removing this covering.
- Using only same-sex care providers and ensuring privacy and confidentiality may help people feel more comfortable while receiving medical care.
- Often people do not understand that sexually transmitted diseases are contracted through sexual activity.
- Women may choose to use birth control, but frequently they will not ask for it or wish to discuss it.
- Under some Pakistani laws, men have different rights than women. For example, women may be severely punished for accusing a man of rape.
- Marriage between cousins is not uncommon and can result in some recessive disorders, such as thalassemia.

- Abortion is generally not considered an acceptable practice.
- Extramarital affairs are sometimes punished severely by law in this country, and women may be persecuted for such activities.
- Premarital sex and pregnancy out of wedlock are sometimes punished by law in Pakistan and are considered taboo.
- Rape is generally thought to bring great shame on the family, and some people prefer that a family member be killed rather than raped.

CHILDREARING
- Male children are generally preferred.
- Many women in Pakistan do not have access to prenatal care, although this is improving.
- Perinatal complications and congenital anomalies are leading causes of death for women and children in this country.
- Female family members usually attend to the laboring mother during childbirth, and fathers are often not present until after the child has been born.
- People present at a birth may not mention the sex of the baby until the placenta has been delivered.
- People may say the call to prayer into the newborn's ear so that it is the first thing the child hears.
- The family may pray immediately after the birth.
- The family may shave the head of the baby at 1 month because they believe the head to be unclean.
- Animal sacrifices are sometimes performed after a birth.
- A bag containing religious verses is sometimes placed around the infant's neck.
- Mothers may breastfeed their infants for up to a few years.

CHILD REARING
- Children attend school for an average of 6–7 years in this country; however, in some parts, females do not attend school at all.

- Families may be ashamed of having a sick child, because this is sometimes thought to reflect the morals of the mother.
- Female children are sometimes raised under stricter rules and are given more discipline than male children.
- The dropout rate for Pakistani girls is about 50%.

FAMILY ROLE

- The family is very important and is the basis for much of a person's identity.
- Male members of the family make most of the family's decisions.
- Elder family members are usually cared for at home and shown great respect.
- Extended family members often live together in a family home.
- Arranged marriages are not uncommon.
- More than half of marriages are between cousins.
- Divorce is relatively uncommon in this country; in urban areas rates are increasing. However, a woman who asks for a divorce may be punished or even killed.

SPIRITUALITY AND BELIEFS

- About 95% of the citizens are Islamic, and the remaining 5% are primarily Christian and Hindu.
- In Pakistan, the Qur'an and Muslim faith guide most life and health-care decisions and practices.
- Muslims pray five times a day facing toward Mecca after washing themselves.
- Organ donation and transplant is a subject of great debate in the Muslim faith: some feel that to remove organs from the body is to mutilate and disrespect a gift from Allah.
- People may wear a small packet of written prayers on their body.

DEATH AND DYING

- In the Muslim religion it is mandated never to give up hope (which may lead to a preference against do-not-resuscitate orders).
- It is generally preferred that the medical provider tell the family first of a poor diagnosis so family members may decide if and when to tell the patient.
- There is likely to be a strong resistance to postmortem examination, because in the Muslim faith the body should be buried intact.
- After death of the patient, the family may wish to wash the body.
- Burial takes place as soon as possible after death—often within 24 hours—and is linked to the timing of daily prayers.

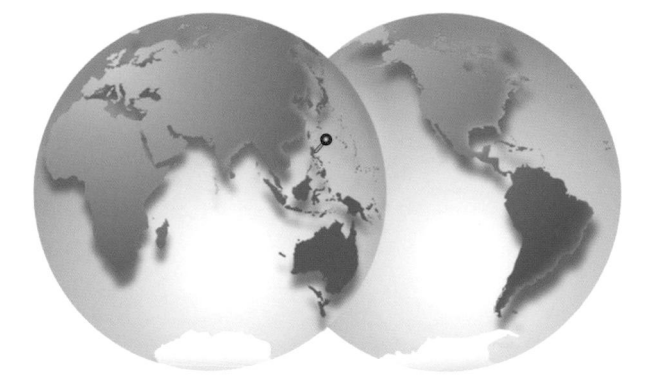

The Philippines

The Republic of the Philippines is a country in Southeast Asia that comprises more than 7000 islands. It has about 92 million people, making it the world's 12th most populated country but just the 47th largest in size. Hence, much of the Philippines is very densely populated, especially because large regions of the terrain are uninhabitable. The earliest human remains are more than 24,000 years old. Different ethnic groups, such as the Negritos—considered to be the oldest group—and the Malayans, migrated there over centuries. In 1521 Ferdinand Magellan arrived, claimed the Philippines for Spain, and established Catholicism and trade. The Spanish controlled the country until 1898, when the United States gained control for $20 million at the end of the Spanish-American War. In 1941, during World War II, Japan invaded the country. During the Japanese occupation, many war crimes were committed, and it is estimated that over a million Filipinos died. This is still a source of anguish for many older Filipinos. In 1945 Allied forces liberated the country, and it was granted its independence.

Today this country is composed of many different ethnicities and cultures. An estimated 11 million Filipinos live outside the Philippines, which is about 11% of its population.

COMMUNICATION
- More than 170 languages are spoken in the Philippines.
- The two national languages are Filipino and English. Many minor languages are also spoken, with Tagalog being the most common indigenous language. It is not unusual for any two people not to speak the same language.
- About 92% of people can read and write in their native language.
- Eye contact is acceptable.
- Personal space is about an arm's length.
- In the Philippines, hand motions to signal "come closer" are used only for animals and are considered insulting to people.
- People may be hesitant to say no and may say yes or remain silent instead of disagreeing.
- Shame is a powerful emotion, and "saving face" is very important. Accusing a patient of not following medical advice or calling attention to a lack of understanding may be considered shameful.
- Avoiding arguments or disagreements is important.

NUTRITION
- People generally eat rice with every meal; main items are roasted pig, salted fish, sausage, chicken, and vegetables cooked in tomato sauce and coconut milk.
- The traditional diet is generally high in sodium from soy sauce, salty cooked meats, sauces, and fast foods.
- Being overweight is generally not considered to be unhealthy and is considered a sign of wealth.
- Rice porridge is often preferred during illnesses.

- Dog meat is considered a delicacy.
- To cure a stomachache, people often toast uncooked rice, add water, and then drink the liquid.
- Alcoholic beverages are popular, including brandy, rum, beer, and *tuba,* which is made from the drippings of a cut palm. Alcohol is not common in Muslim areas.
- Other popular beverages include tea, coffee, and fruit and soft drinks.
- Many people are lactose-intolerant.
- About 28 million Filipinos are unable to buy enough food, and about a third of young children are underweight.
- Vitamin A deficiencies and iron deficiency anemia are common problems.

PHYSICAL ILLNESS
- People may wait until an illness is advanced before seeking treatment.
- Hepatitis B is a common disease in this country and is transmitted by sexual contact, contact with other body fluids, and from an infected mother to her infant.
- There have been outbreaks of Ebola, meningitis, and severe acute respiratory syndrome in the Philippines in recent years.
- People may be resistant to oxygen delivery because they believe it indicates their condition is very serious.
- In the hospital, people may feel uncomfortable going out of their room because of modesty.
- Regular bowel movements are considered important for health.
- Respiratory tract conditions are the primary cause of death in this country, including lower respiratory tract infections, tuberculosis, and chronic obstructive pulmonary disease.
- Cardiovascular disease is another major cause of death.
- Diarrheal diseases are a common cause of death.
- Diabetes is another leading cause of death and often goes undiagnosed or untreated.

- Malaria and other parasitic infections are common in the Philippines.
- Violence is a major cause of death in this country, primarily due to assaults, gang violence, and political turmoil in some regions.
- Obesity is a growing problem in this country; however, rates are still lower than in many more developed countries.
- Sponge baths are preferred by some Filipino patients because showers are thought to cause arthritis.
- Having the shower and the toilet in the same room is considered by some to be unhygienic.
- The need to ambulate after surgery and during illness may not be well received by patients because they believe that rest is most important.

MENTAL ILLNESS
- Mental illnesses are often thought to result from witchcraft or demons and are often associated with shame and stigmatization for the whole family.
- Mental health treatment is largely unavailable in this country aside from a few inpatient facilities, which are often overcrowded and have limited resources.
- "Soul loss" is believed to occur when the soul leaves the body because of fear, shock, or desire and requires prayer, fasting, and possibly an exorcism.
- The abuse of methamphetamines as well as of other illegal drugs is a major problem in this country.
- Alcoholism is often not taken seriously; however, rates are believed to be relatively low.

PAIN
- Pain is sometimes considered the "will of God" and therefore to be endured, not expressed.
- People may prefer intravenous and oral pain medications to intramuscular medications.

SEXUALITY

■ Homosexuality is generally tolerated.

■ The rhythm method of birth control is the only birth control in this country due to the influences of the Catholic church.

■ Divorce is not legal; even if the marriage and divorce take place in another country, the divorce is still not considered legal.

■ Spousal abuse is a common problem and is often ignored.

■ Women may not seek medical care due to modesty and may prefer same-sex providers.

CHILDBEARING

■ Perinatal deaths are a major problem.

■ Prenatal care is provided to about 90% of women, but skilled birth attendants are present at only about 60% of births.

■ Iron deficiency anemia is a common problem in pregnant women.

■ People believe that a pregnant mother's food cravings must be satisfied or they will hurt the baby.

■ Prenatal vitamins are sometimes thought to harm the baby.

■ Vaginal deliveries are generally preferred.

■ The grandmother instead of the father may attend the delivery and be with the mother.

■ During the birth the father may remain at work or go out with his friends.

■ It may be preferred that any issues with the baby be discussed first with the father.

■ Filipino families often do not circumcise their children at or near the time of birth.

CHILD REARING

■ The average child attends school for 12 years in this country.

■ Breastfeeding is common and may last until the child is around 2 years old.

- People believe the "evil eye" is a curse caused by compliments to the child and by envy; it is believed to make a child ill. The curse may be neutralized by making a cross on the child's forehead with saliva on the finger.
- Children are often raised using fear, shame, and teasing to motivate them to have good behavior.
- Males are often circumcised at around 12 years of age, generally in a ritual where the foreskin is pulled and then cut without anesthesia.
- Children often live with their parents into adulthood.
- Education, valuing family, respect for elders, and success are common values taught to children.

FAMILY ROLE

- People are very loyal to their family members, and elders are shown great respect.
- The husband is the head of the family, but the wife often has equal authority on such issues as finances and child rearing.
- A female relative may stay with an ill family member throughout a hospitalization.
- The children are expected to care for their aging parents at home.
- Some older family members may not want to be a burden to their family and will not seek health care due to this fear.
- Some Muslim Filipino families practice polygamy.
- The oldest child is often put through school with the aid of the family. The family may then expect that each successive child is to be helped financially by the elder sibling.

SPIRITUALITY AND BELIEFS

- 80% of Filipinos are Roman Catholic, 9% are Protestant, and 6% are Muslim.
- An individual may follow Catholicism as well as mysticism.
- Patients often wear rosaries, medals, and other religious jewelry to promote healing.

- Many people wear a small maroon bag around their neck for healing and will be resistant to taking it off.
- Aromatherapy and having a pleasant body odor are generally very important to people.
- Exercise, especially walking, is believed to be an important part of health.

DEATH AND DYING

- Organ donation is not common.
- Family members may want to be told about a poor prognosis before the patient is told. The family may believe that telling the patient only increases the patient's suffering.
- Roman Catholics generally want to have last rites performed by a priest near the time of death.
- Family members may want to wash the body before it is transported.
- Families may be very resistant to stopping life support.

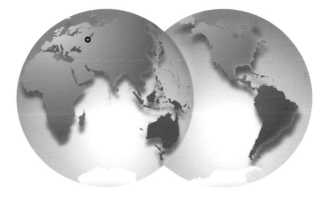

Russia

Russia, or the Russian Federation, is located in Northern Eurasia and is the largest country in terms of land mass; it occupies one-ninth of the world's land mass. Russia is the ninth largest country in terms of population, with a total of 142 million people. The region was developed by the Finno-Ugric peoples and Eastern Slavs between the 3rd and 8th centuries. In 988, Christianity was adopted from the Byzantines. The civilization began to blend the Slavic culture with Orthodox Christianity, both of which have been defining forces throughout much of Russia's history. In the 15th century, Ivan III, or Ivan the Great, united Russia under one ruling government and created the role of Tsar. The Russian Revolution of 1917 was led by Vladimir Lenin and ended in the imprisonment of the last Tsar, Nicholas II. After a civil war, the Bolshevik party emerged victorious and created the Union of Soviet Socialist Republics (USSR). Joseph Stalin was elected after Lenin died in 1924 and further strengthened the ruling communist party. Russia remained a closed communist country until December 1991, when the USSR was dissolved. The country became the Russian Federation and drafted a new constitution in 1993. Since then, Russia has struggled to establish economic and political stability.

COMMUNICATION
■ The primary language of Russia is Russian, but a few minor languages are also spoken, such as Tatar and Ukrainian.
■ Almost all people can read and write in their native language.
■ Handshakes are appropriate greetings and are often very firm.
■ Direct eye contact is considered acceptable.
■ Personal space is very close.
■ Standing with the hands in one's pockets is considered rude.
■ Smiling a great deal can be considered phony and silly.
■ Proper titles, such as Miss., Mrs. and Mr., are appreciated when addressing Russians.
■ High-tech medical equipment is often not well understood and should be explained.
■ Some people are afraid of answering questions due to a lifetime of strict political supervision.
■ In Russia, it is often necessary to bribe health-care providers to receive good care. This may influence the way Russians communicate with health-care workers.

NUTRITION
■ Traditional Russian foods include poultry, pork, fish, cabbage, potatoes, and breads. Bread is a symbol of hospitality.
■ Some northern regions of Russia have very long cold winters with short growing seasons. Fresh fruits and vegetables may be limited in these areas.
■ In Russia, lunch is often the largest meal of the day.
■ Fast foods are popular in Russia.

- The typical Russian diet is high in starch, sodium, and fat.
- Soups are an important part of Russian cuisine and are generally preferred during times of illness.
- Russia is one of the largest consumers of tea in the world, with black tea and green tea being the most popular.
- Ice is not generally put into beverages.
- Alcohol is commonly served at meals, with vodka being the most popular traditional Russian beverage. Beer is the second most popular drink in Russia, followed by wine.
- The Russian diet has been shown to be low in antioxidants, especially vitamin C, folic acid, and selenium. Iron deficiency anemia is also common.
- It is believed that cold beverages should be avoided during illness.

PHYSICAL ILLNESS
- People may believe that taking too many medications can cause illnesses.
- About 1.2% of Russians are HIV-positive, a percentage that has doubled in the past 10 years.
- In Russia it is a common concern that the blood supply for blood transplants is contaminated with AIDS or other diseases.
- The most common cause of death in Russia is cardiovascular disease.
- Poisoning, primarily from alcohol, is the third most common cause of death in Russia.
- Self-inflicted injuries, violence, and road traffic accidents are three other leading causes of death. These are thought to result from high rates of alcoholism.
- Stomach, colon, and rectal cancer are other common causes of death and have been shown to be related to alcohol abuse.
- Cirrhosis of the liver is the 10th most common cause of death, resulting from alcoholism and hepatitis infections.

- The most common types of cancer are trachea, bronchus, and lung, which are linked to high rates of smoking.
- About 50% of Russian adults smoke cigarettes.
- Obesity rates in Russia are thought to be comparable to those of the United States; there is little research on the subject because Russians define obesity differently.
- Russians may believe that ambulating during illness or recovery is unhealthy and may be resistant.
- Staying warm during illnesses is thought to be very important, and patients may wear layers with their hospital gowns.
- Uninterrupted sleep is considered especially important.
- Russians often do not wash their hair during illnesses.
- Cupping, which involves heating a cup or bowl and placing it against the skin to create suction, is believed to pull out the illness. This process sometimes leaves a scar.
- Mustard paste is often rubbed on the chest to cure respiratory illnesses.
- Mustard plasters are a poultice made of mustard seeds that are applied to the back and chest to help in recovery.

MENTAL ILLNESS
- Mental illness is very stigmatized.
- Mental health care is generally reserved for acute mental illnesses; other mental health problems are largely untreated.
- In Russia, mental illnesses are often treated with sedatives.
- Russians are generally not comfortable talking about their problems and feelings.
- Mental health treatment in the United States is very different from treatments in Russia and may not be understood by patients and their families.
- There are very high rates of alcohol abuse, with an estimated 10 million alcoholics in Russia.

- In this country, children often begin drinking and smoking at age 7 years.
- There are three to five million drug addicts in Russia, with popular drugs being cannabis, opioids, and cocaine.
- Political refugees may feel a great deal of fear, anxiety, and guilt for those they have left behind.

PAIN
- Russians may have a high pain threshold; they may be stoic and not express their pain.
- Pain medication is generally well received.

SEXUALITY
- Modesty is important, and sex is not openly discussed, even in families.
- Sex education is not taught in schools in Russia, and parents often do not teach their children about sex.
- Homosexuality is not accepted.
- Extramarital affairs are common in Russia for both men and women.
- Abortion is legal in Russia and, although it is very common, it is not discussed openly.
- In Russia 28 of 1000 pregnancies are to unwed teenage mothers. This is the second highest rate of teenage pregnancies in developed nations in the world, behind the United States.
- In Russia, birth control is very expensive and is not commonly used.
- HIV rates are on the rise in this country. This is thought to result from intravenous drug abuse rates and sex during intoxication.
- Some members of the Russian Orthodox Church do not believe in birth control.

CHILDBEARING

- Birth rates are very low in Russia, with 1.4 births per woman. Because of this, the population of Russia is shrinking, and national campaigns are attempting to increase the birth rate.

- In Russia prenatal care is provided early in a pregnancy, and significant information is generally shared between clinics.

- Russians may believe that lifting items or skipping stairs causes the cord to drape around the baby's neck or the baby to be breech.

- It is generally believed that telling an expecting mother bad news is very bad for the pregnancy.

- It is thought that too much light in the delivery room hurts the baby's eyes.

- In Russia usually only female family members are present in the delivery room.

- Breastfeeding is common and valued.

- In Russia the mother and the baby usually stay in the hospital for a week.

- A newborn baby may be shown only to the birth attendants and the father for 1 month because of fears about a curse being placed on the baby.

- All gifts purchased for a baby should be purchased after the baby is born to avoid bad luck.

CHILD REARING

- The average child in Russia begins school at age 7 and attends school for 10 to 11 years.

- Children are often very protected as they are frequently single children and are raised in a home with their parents and grandparents.

- Parents in Russia often have to be strong advocates for their children and may feel that they need to insist on more thorough medical testing and treatment.
- Parents are generally proud of their children but may be concerned that too many compliments will bring about an "evil eye" curse.
- Parents teach their children to value education and family.

FAMILY ROLE

- The decision making for the family is often done by the dominant person, which may be any family member, or jointly by the husband and wife.
- The common family unit is the extended family.
- Domestic violence is common and is thought to be related to alcohol abuse. Domestic violence is often ignored and treatment is limited.
- Women are generally expected to care for their children and husband, run the home, and earn a living, and this is believed to have resulted in the current low birth rates.
- Grandparents or other relatives often care for the children while the mother works.
- Adult family members are expected to take elderly family members into their home and care for them.

SPIRITUALITY AND BELIEFS

- 63% of Russians are Russian Orthodox Christians, 16% are nonbelievers, 12% are believers but do not practice any faith, 6% are Muslim, and about 1% are Buddhist, Jewish, or other.
- Some people believe that withholding emotions and "being strong" are important.
- Relaxation is thought to be important to health.
- It is believed that sitting on a cold surface, such as the ground, is hazardous to a female's health and reproductive organs.

■ It is considered bad luck to step over a person or any part of a person as this will cause that individual to stop growing.

DEATH AND DYING
■ People generally prefer to die at home.
■ Visitors sometimes believe that it is important to be cheerful to avoid upsetting a patient.
■ Do-not-resuscitate orders are often accepted.
■ Family members may want to wash the patient's body after death.
■ Autopsy is not generally acceptable.

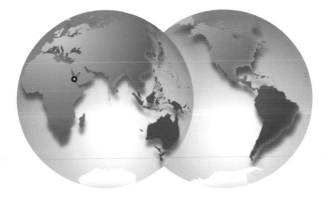

Saudi Arabia

The Kingdom of Saudi Arabia is a country located on the Arabian Peninsula. The country encompasses approximately 2,150,000 square miles, making it the largest country in the Middle East and the 14th largest country in the world. Saudi Arabia has a population of approximately 28 million people, making it the world's 46th most populous country. Saudi Arabia is also referred to as "The Land of the Two Holy Mosques" as it is home to the two holiest places in Islam, Mecca and Medina.

The territory of modern-day Saudi Arabia has been inhabited for more than 5000 years. The country's more recent history is commonly associated with the rise of the Saudi dynasty in the mid-1700s. Since that time, rule by the family of Saud has gone through various periods of rise and decline. In 1932 various regions on the peninsula were unified as the Kingdom of Saudi Arabia.

Saudi Arabia is a theocratic Islamic state and a monarchy ruled by King Abdullah bin Abdul-Aziz. The country is the world's largest exporter of petroleum, which provides the government with great wealth but also vulnerability to fluctuations in global oil prices. About 23% of the population in Saudi Arabia is composed of foreign workers, primarily from Asia and Africa.

COMMUNICATION

- The official language of Saudi Arabia is Arabic.
- About 84% of men and 70% of women can read and write in their native language.
- Men may shake hands with right hand. Women are not introduced, and they may not want to be touched or offered a handshake.
- People may not be comfortable with direct eye contact with persons of the opposite sex.
- The male head of the family may speak for all women in his household and act as the family decision maker.
- It is often beneficial to ask the male head of the household how to address the family member who is the patient and what name should be used.
- Families may be assertive about getting good health care, and the patient may take a passive roll.
- People may be more willing to share information if the health-care provider shares personal information first.
- Same-sex adults may hold hands while talking and walking together.

NUTRITION

- Unleavened bread, called *khobz,* is served with almost all meals; rice, lamb, chicken, and falafel (fried chickpeas) are common foods.
- Fast foods are very popular in Saudi Arabia.
- Tea is important; it is served black and comes in many flavors.
- Arabic coffee accompanied with dates is also popular and traditionally served in the home when guests visit.

- Fasting is important to Muslims and involves not eating, drinking, or smoking until sundown on certain days of the year.
- *Halal* meat is from animals that are slaughtered in a certain way and may be important to Muslims.
- The Muslim practice of abstaining from alcohol is observed by most Saudi Arabians.
- Being overweight may be considered healthy in this country.
- Malnutrition is present in around 10% of children in this country; however, obesity, diabetes, and hypertension are a growing problem in the adult population.
- It is traditional for family members to bring sweets to ill family members.

PHYSICAL ILLNESS
- Saudi Arabians have one of the highest rates of type II diabetes in the world due to being sedentary, changing eating habits, and adopting the Western lifestyle.
- Diabetes and related cardiac, renal, and eye complications are a major cause of morbidity and mortality in Saudi Arabia.
- Sickle cell anemia occurs mainly in the eastern part of Saudi Arabia.
- Cardiovascular disease is the primary cause of death in this country.
- Lower respiratory infections, nephritis, and nephrosis are other major causes of death in this country.
- In Saudi Arabia, about 34% of men older than 12 years smoke cigarettes.
- Congenital anomalies are problematic in Saudi Arabia, the most common being those of the central nervous system (such as spina bifida) and cardiovascular (such as cardiac septal defects and tetralogy of Fallot).
- Motor vehicle accidents are one of the major causes of death and injury in Saudi Arabia.
- Female patients and their husbands may refuse care if it requires a woman to be seen undressed by any male other than her husband.

MENTAL ILLNESS

■ People may believe that counseling is unnecessary because problems can and should be solved within the family. Tribal elders may also sometimes be consulted to provide some form of counseling.

■ Traditional medicine may include exorcism, which attempts to rid the person of evil spirits.

■ Because of the stigma associated with mental illnesses, an illness may be very advanced before the patient is brought in for treatment.

■ Psychiatric medications that are common in some countries are becoming more common in Saudi Arabia.

PAIN

■ People may be very expressive about their pain.

■ Some Muslims believe that pain is "Allah's will" and should not be treated with pain relievers.

■ Intoxicating pain relievers are believed by some to be amoral.

■ Nonpharmaceutical remedies include massage therapy, cupping, and acupuncture.

SEXUALITY

■ Traditional Saudi dress adheres to principles of modesty. Women may cover most of their body (including the hair) in public. Men traditionally wear a loose-fitting ankle-length garment called a *thobes.*

■ Female providers may be preferred for women's care.

■ The male partner is usually the one to determine if contraception will be used.

■ Female purity, modesty, and sexual segregation are all reflections of family honor.

■ Menstruating women are considered unclean and do not pray or fast.

■ Marriages are often arranged.

■ Arranged meetings between potential dating partners are often done with a chaperone present.

- Rape is very shameful for the woman and her family but is often underreported.
- Abortions are legal only to protect the life of the mother and must be co-authorized by three physicians.
- Adultery is sometimes severely punished by law in this country.

CHILDBEARING
- A pregnant mother is usually given whatever foods she desires.
- Male children are generally preferred.
- Childbearing education classes are not common.
- A woman may be under pressure from her husband and extended family until she gives birth to a son.
- Saudi Arabia has had high rates of babies born with congenital anomalies due to marriages between cousins and genetic predispositions, although prenatal testing has reduced numbers in recent years.
- Rosemary and thyme teas are thought to increase contractions.
- Mothers may be very vocal and expressive during deliveries.
- Fathers are generally not present at the birth in this country; instead, a female family member assists the mother.
- The family may want to bury the placenta, although this is less common for hospital births.
- Traditionally, a new mother has a period of rest for 40 days after birth.

CHILD REARING
- The average child attends school for about 15 years in this country, before entering college or a vocation.
- Breastfeeding is generally accepted.
- Male circumcision is common.
- The mother is usually responsible for most of the parental duties.
- Parents tend to be permissive with small children and become more strict as the child matures.

- Girls and boys generally have equal educational opportunities, although girls may be restricted from studying some "male" subjects, such as engineering.
- When raising children, emphasis is usually placed on faith and the value of the family's reputation.

FAMILY ROLE

- Family honor is extremely important.
- A family member or paid family representative usually remains with a patient.
- Some husbands may not allow their wives to sign a consent form.
- The eldest son is usually given most of the family's inheritance.
- Elders are generally cared for at home by the family.
- Domestic violence is a problem, but it is not a topic of open discussion and is often not reported.
- Divorce and remarriage have been much stigmatized, but they are becoming more common and accepted.

SPIRITUALITY AND BELIEFS

- Almost everyone in Saudi Arabia is reported to be a Muslim.
- Muslims pray five times a day facing Mecca, a city in Saudi Arabia and the holiest meeting site in the Muslim faith.
- Allah controls everything; Muslims may feel that certain issues should not be discussed because they are in "Allah's hands."
- Family and children with genetic defects are sometimes seen as tests of faith and endurance.

DEATH AND DYING

- People may be very hesitant to sign a do-not-resuscitate order and may not wish even to discuss it because it is seen as going against their religious belief not to give up hope.

- Organ donation may not be well received due to the Muslim principle that the body should be buried intact, although donation is becoming more common in some parts of the country.
- Autopsy may not be well received due to the desire in this culture for a rapid burial.
- Burial by sunset on the day of the death may be desired and timed relative to daily prayers.
- Male members of the family may be the only people who will discuss death or serious illness.
- Women may be very vocal during their grieving.
- The body of the deceased may be washed, perfumed, and dressed in a white garment.

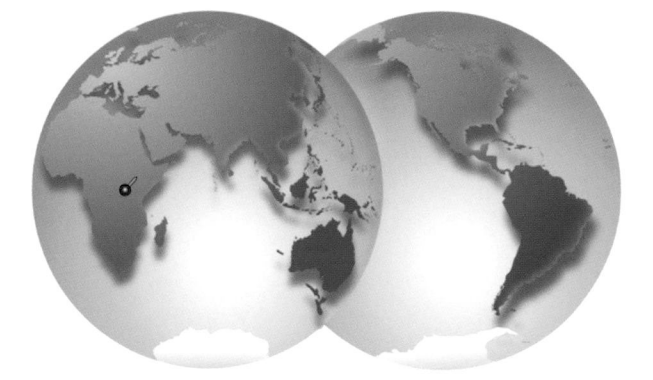

Uganda

The Republic of Uganda is a land-locked nation in East Africa. The population of Uganda is more than 32 million and is growing rapidly due to its fertility rate of almost seven children per woman. This is the third highest birth rate in the world. The population of Uganda is also very young, with a median age of 15 years. The land size of this country is about 236,000 square miles, making it the 81st largest country in the world. Half the population lives below the international poverty line. In recent decades, HIV has become a major problem. Nevertheless, Uganda has been one of the few countries to lower its rates of HIV infections significantly. This major accomplishment was achieved through a national and international effort to educate people and provide protection and testing to prevent the spread of HIV.

Uganda is a presidential republic with a multiparty system. In the last few decades, Uganda has had to cope with conflict from the neighboring Democratic Republic of Congo and with long-running civil guerilla conflict fought by the Lord's Resistance Army in the north of the country. Despite such domestic troubles, Uganda is active in regional organizations, such as the African Union, and has participated in activities such as peacekeeping in Somalia. Uganda's economy has also seen robust growth in the last few years, despite the global economic recession.

COMMUNICATION
- The national language of Uganda is English; however, about 40 languages are also in regular use, which reflects the numerous ethnic groups.
- Luganda is the most commonly spoken local language, followed by Lusoga and Runy Ankore.
- About 67% of people can read or write in their native language.
- People from Uganda generally greet each other by shaking hands.
- Personal space is limited. People conversing generally have less than an arm's length between them.
- People of the same sex frequently touch, especially hands and arms. People of the opposite sex do not usually touch, with the exception of shaking hands.
- People of different genders usually do not make eye contact. As a sign of respect, young people do not look their elders in the eye.
- Physicians and nurses are highly respected.
- People are sometimes intimidated by the act of seeking medical care.
- Pointing a finger is considered rude.

NUTRITION
- Traditional foods in Uganda include corn meal, beans, potatoes, millet, cassava, bananas, and meat. Meat is rarely eaten in more rural and poor areas.
- About one-fourth of the population is malnourished; this rate does not show indications of improving.

■ The average diet in this country often does not contain enough protein and may lead to health problems, such as kwashiorkor and marasmus.

■ Water is piped into urban areas of Uganda; however, it must be boiled before it is suitable for drinking. In rural areas, people often get their water from protected wells or boreholes, which are usually safe, or from streams and rivers, which are often contaminated with bacteria, parasites, and other pollutants.

PHYSICAL ILLNESS

■ More than half of the population lives in malarial areas and is exposed to malaria throughout the year. Malaria is the leading cause of death in this country.

■ Malaria is generally most serious in children younger than 5 years, pregnant women, and individuals with HIV.

■ Currently, 6.7% of Ugandans are infected with HIV and AIDS. This is down from about 15% in 1991, when the rate peaked.

■ HIV is still responsible for significant morbidity and mortality rates in Uganda and is the second leading cause of death.

■ Infectious diseases, such as lower respiratory infections, diarrheal diseases, tuberculosis, and measles, are among the leading causes of death.

■ Water-borne illnesses are a common problem in Uganda due to poor water sanitation. The illnesses cause dysentery and diarrhea, which often present as severe and chronic diarrhea.

■ In recent years, there have been outbreaks of Ebola virus in some regions of Uganda.

■ Marburg's hemorrhagic fever has been recorded in Uganda in recent years.

■ Sickle cell anemia is a fairly common disease. Affected individuals are generally given folic acid and prophylactic antimalarial treatment.

■ Uganda families have very limited access to medications and may split prescriptions among family members, which often results in no one receiving a complete therapeutic dose.

- Uganda has many traditional practices that offer various treatment modalities. One example involves cutting open the skin, putting herbs or animal horns into the cut, and then sucking the blood from the wound.

MENTAL ILLNESS

- Mental illnesses are often considered as bringing shame to the patient and the entire family.
- In some portions of this population, mental illnesses are believed to run in families, which can lead to the belief that the other family members are also mentally ill.
- People diagnosed with mental health illnesses are often abandoned by their families.
- This country, particularly the northern region, has experienced a great deal of turmoil, and many people suffer from post-traumatic stress disorder.
- Depression is believed to result from problems between the living and the dead.
- A small number of people with mental health issues in Uganda participate in group therapy and counseling, but psychiatric medications are even less common.
- There are very few psychiatrists in Uganda, and the few who practice are primarily in the urban areas.
- Tobacco is used heavily in this country, especially by men.
- Homemade alcohol is commonly abused.

PAIN

- Ugandans may believe that pain is good during an illness or a treatment because it means the patient is healing.
- Men may hide their pain to attempt to appear stoic.
- Ugandans generally accept the use of pain medications.

- Acupuncture is a common and accepted method of pain management because it is available to rural healers.
- Palliative care and pain management are becoming more available in many urban hospitals and health centers.

SEXUALITY

- Uganda has promoted the "ABC plan" to reduce HIV rates: Abstinence, Be faithful, and use Condoms.
- Female genital mutilation is still practiced usually in rural areas, primarily in tribal groups living along the eastern border.
- Due to the lack of perinatal care in Uganda, women who endure difficult deliveries may have long-term complications with their reproductive organs.
- Because of Uganda's aggressive fight against AIDS, condoms are used frequently.
- Women may believe that using birth control will make them permanently infertile.
- Women do not frequently use modern methods of family planning.
- Rates of unwanted pregnancies and pregnancies in unwed mothers are high in this country because of Ugandan women's distrust of contraceptives and lack of access to them.
- About one in five pregnancies in this country ends in abortion, many of which are performed unsafely.
- Many women who have abortions in this country have complications from the procedure.
- Men may have multiple families or partners, and polygamy is still an acceptable practice in many areas.
- Homosexuality is illegal in Uganda; proposed legislation could result in the death penalty for homosexuals and prosecution for anyone who knows a homosexual and does not report the person to the authorities.

CHILDBEARING

- Perinatal deaths are the fifth highest cause of death in Uganda.
- Uganda has a high rate of infant and maternal deaths from complications during childbirth. As a result of this knowledge, laboring women may be very fearful.
- Male children are generally preferred.
- Breastfeeding is generally believed to be a form of birth control, even though it does not protect against pregnancy.

CHILD REARING

- Children in Uganda attend school for an average of 10 years.
- There are nearly two million orphans in Uganda who have lost their parents to AIDS; many of these children are also infected.
- Some families use aggressive physical punishment to discipline their children.
- Uganda has some guerilla groups that kidnap children and force them to become soldiers for their cause. Many children walk several miles from their villages to a safe place every night to avoid being kidnapped.
- Uganda has very high rates of malaria, which is often most severe in children.
- Older children often help raise their younger siblings, which may result in their maturing at a young age.

FAMILY ROLE

- Many households in Uganda have lost a family member to AIDS. There are many single-parent households, and many children have been orphaned after the death of both parents.
- Men from this country may have more than one family or wife.
- Often when someone dies, another person will be assigned to fill the role of the deceased family member.
- If a woman does not give birth to a male child, it is generally believed that the father can then have children with another woman.

- Grandparents frequently raise grandchildren who have lost their parents to AIDS.
- Elderly family members have traditionally been cared for at home by their children, but due to high rates of AIDS, poverty, and turmoil, this has become less common, leaving older people to care for themselves.

SPIRITUALITY AND BELIEFS

- In Uganda, about 42% are Roman Catholic, another 42% are Christian, and 12% are Muslim.
- Deceased ancestors are believed to communicate with the living and influence their daily lives.
- Elders are highly respected, and it is thought that an illness can result as punishment by an ancestral spirit for disrespect of an elder.
- Human sacrifices, frequently children, are increasing in Uganda, as some people believe this will help them achieve wealth and prosperity.
- Traditional healers are common and often prescribe natural and spiritual remedies.

DEATH AND DYING

- The life expectancy in Uganda is 52 years, mostly due to HIV/AIDS.
- Women tend to be very expressive in their grief.
- People generally prefer to die at home.
- Neighbors and friends may stigmatize the home of a dying person because they believe the family has done something wrong or may infect them as well.
- Organ donation and autopsies are generally not considered acceptable.
- Do-not-resuscitate orders are not common or well understood in Uganda because of the lack of available services and organized practices.

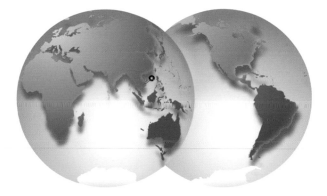

Vietnam

The Socialist Republic of Vietnam is a small country located on a peninsula in Southeast Asia, just south of China. Vietnam is the world's 13th most populated country, with 86 million people, and the 65th largest in land mass. Vietnam broke away from China in 938 and was independent until it was colonized by the French in the mid-19th century. After the French were expelled in the mid-20th century, the country was divided. The United States became involved in the fighting between North and South Vietnam, with the North Vietnamese eventually winning the war and creating communist Vietnam. Vietnam was a closed communist country until 1986, when it began to focus on economic development and reestablishing international diplomatic relationships. Vietnam has a successfully growing economy and is a member of the World Trade Organization and the United Nations Security Council.

COMMUNICATION

- The primary language of Vietnam is Vietnamese, with English being a common second language.
- It is generally acceptable to greet someone with a handshake or by bowing the head.
- Proper titles are appreciated when addressing Vietnamese, such as Miss, Mrs., Ms., and Mr., followed by the first or last name.
- People generally do not make eye contact while conversing and often look down instead.
- To blink the eyes means that a message has been received.
- People prefer a large area of personal space.
- People may introduce themselves with their last name first, their middle name second, and their first name last.
- It is common for people to not express their feelings or emotions when communicating.
- It is considered disrespectful to position oneself higher than the oldest member of the family.
- Detailed information and health teaching is generally well received by patients and family members.
- The oldest male in the family often makes all the decisions for the family.

NUTRITION

- Rice is a staple as are certain meats, vegetables, French bread, and noodles.
- Soft, warm foods are considered appropriate for ill people.
- Iced beverages are not generally accepted.
- Lactose intolerance is common in the Vietnamese population.

PHYSICAL ILLNESS

- The primary fatal disease in Vietnam is cardiovascular, followed by chronic obstructive pulmonary disease and respiratory infections including tuberculosis.

- People may be embarrassed by vomiting and may deny emesis or try to cover it up.
- People are often particularly uncomfortable discussing bowel habits or problems, and it is sometimes difficult to obtain information about these issues.
- In Vietnam the head is believed to hold the soul, therefore, it is best to ask permission before touching a patient's head.
- Health maintenance is not well understood in this country, and patients often do not seek treatment until they are experiencing significant symptoms.
- Cupping is a common practice: a bowl or cup is placed on the skin and heated to produce suction on this skin. Cupping is thought to pull out the bad energy that is making the person ill. This practice often leaves a bruise on the skin.
- Coining is a practice in which a coin or other solid object is rubbed repeatedly on the skin to extract bad energy or air that is making the person ill. This practice may leave a bruise or abrasion on the skin.
- Vietnam has had several recent outbreaks of avian influenza and severe acute respiratory syndrome.
- There is much trauma due to motor scooter accidents and physical combat, especially between young males.

MENTAL ILLNESS
- There is a social stigmatization associated with mental illness, and therefore patients often wait until symptoms are severe before seeking treatment.
- People may believe that mental illnesses are due to a lack of spiritual harmony in the affected individual or by the ancestors of the person coming back to visit.

PAIN
- People are generally tolerant of pain and may even try to smile or appear happy in an attempt to hide their pain.

■ Warm compresses are thought to be beneficial and are appreciated during times of discomfort or pain.

SEXUALITY
■ In many families, males are valued more than females.
■ Women's breasts and torso are regarded as very private and should be covered as much as possible.
■ Same-sex care providers are preferred.
■ Pregnancies in unwed mothers are considered shameful, and many women try herbs to induce an abortion.
■ Significant regular menstrual flow is considered healthy, which sometimes causes an issue with those birth-control methods that decrease the menstrual flow.
■ Domestic violence is an accepted practice in some parts of this culture.

CHILDBEARING
■ During childbirth, women want warm liquids and to be kept warm with lots of clothing, blankets, and socks regardless of the actual temperature.
■ Women may not ask many questions or show their pain or fear; however, providing them information and reassurance can be helpful.
■ Women are generally the primary caregivers during deliveries, but the father may attend the birth.
■ Breastfeeding is an acceptable and common practice.

CHILD REARING
■ Circumcision is an acceptable practice.
■ Children are considered to be 1 year old at birth.
■ It is very important that children do not shame the family.
■ Primarily through role modeling, children are taught to be honest, quiet, and polite.

FAMILY ROLE
- The eldest male is generally the head of the family.
- Elders are highly regarded and are treated with the utmost respect.
- The family unit in Vietnam is the extended family.
- Eastern and herbal remedies are a major part of heath care.
- If the parents have other jobs or duties, family elders are often expected to provide care for the children and cook for the family.

SPIRITUALITY AND BELIEFS
- Buddhism and Catholicism are the two main religions in this country.
- Some people believe that illnesses are a punishment for bad deeds or behaviors.
- Many people believe in reincarnation, so death is thought to be a way to elevate a person to a better life.

DEATH AND DYING
- People believe that placing rice, coins, or jewels in the mouth of the deceased may help the person travel after death.
- Catholics often wish to have a priest present at the time of death to say last rights for the dying person.
- Buddhists have a death ritual that may last for several days that involves praying and burning incense.
- Organ donation or autopsies are not common practices.

Tools

STANDARD-TO-METRIC CONVERSIONS

WEIGHT		TEMP		HEIGHT	
lb	**kg**	**°F**	**°C**	**in**	**cm**
325	148	212	100 (boil)	56	142
300	136	107	42.2	57	145
275	125	106	41.6	58	147
250	114	105	40.6	59	150
225	102	104	40.0	60	152
210	96	103	39.4	61	155
200	91	102	38.9	62	157
190	86	101	38.3	63	160
180	82	100	37.8	64	163
170	77	99	37.2	65	165
160	73	**98.6**	**37.0**	66	168
150	68	98	36.7	67	170
140	64	97	36.1	68	173
130	59	96	35.6	69	175
120	55	95	35.0	70	178
110	50	94	34.4	71	180
100	46	93	34.0	72	183
90	41	92	33.3	73	185
80	36	91	32.8	74	188
70	32	90	32.1	75	191

STANDARD-TO-METRIC CONVERSIONS—Cont'd

WEIGHT		TEMP		HEIGHT	
lb	kg	°F	°C	in	cm
60	27	32	0 (freeze)	76	193
50	23			77	196
40	18			78	199
30	14				
25	11				
20	9				
15	7				
10	4.5				
5	2.3				

COMMON EQUIVALENTS

VOL		WEIGHT	
1 cc	1 mL	1 mg	1000 mcg
1 tsp	5 mL	1 g	1000 mg
1 tbsp	15 mL	1 kg	1000 gram
1 oz	30 mL	1 grain	60 mg
1 cup	240 mL	1/150 grain	0.4 mg
1 pint	473 mL	1 kg	2.2 lb
1 quart	946 mL	1 L of fluid	1 kg
1 liter	33.5960 oz	1 oz	28 g

COMMON CONVERSION FORMULAS

	STANDARD	METRIC
Wt	lb = kg × 2.2	kg = lb × 0.45 (lb ÷ 2) − 10%
Temp	°F = (°C × 1.8) + 32	°C = (°F − 32) × 0.556
Vol	oz to mL = oz × 30	mL to oz = mL ÷ 30
Length	in = cm × 0.394	cm = in × 2.54

BODY SURFACE AREA

CM AND KG	IN. AND LB
$\sqrt{[(\text{height} \times \text{weight}) \div 3600]}$	$\sqrt{[(\text{height} \times \text{weight}) \div 3131]}$

Waist-to-Hip Ratio

- Measure circumference of waist at its narrowest point with stomach relaxed.
- Measure circumference of hips at fullest point where buttocks protrude most.
- Divide circumference of waist by circumference of hips.

Women should have a waist-to-hip ratio ≤0.8.

Men should have a waist-to-hip ratio ≤0.95

Frequently Used Phone Numbers

Overhead Code: _____

Security: _____

Admitting: _____

Blood Bank: _____

Burn Unit: _____

CICU (CCU): _____

Chaplain/Pastor: _____

Computer Help: _____

CT: _____

Dietary/Dietitian: _____

ECG: 12-Lead: _____

Emergency: _____

Intensive Care Unit: _____

Interpreter Services: _____

Laboratory: _____

Maintenance-Engineering: _____

Med-Surg: _____

MRI: _____

Nutrition: Food Services: _____

Occupational Therapy: _____

PACU (Recovery): _____

Pediatrics: _____

Pharmacy: _____
Physical Therapy: _____
Respiratory: _____
Social Services: _____
Speech-Language Pathology: _____
Supervisor/Manager: _____
Surgery: Day/Outpatient: _____
Surgery: Inpatient: _____
Telemetry Unit: _____
X-Ray: _____

Poison Control (National)	800-222-1222	_____
Chemtrec (HazMat; 24-hr)	800-424-9300	_____
CDC (Biological; 24-hr)	770-488-7100	_____
Divers Alert Network	919-684-8111	_____
USAMRIID (Biological)	888-872-7443	_____
REAC/TS (Radiation)	423-576-3131	_____

Consent

■ **Informed:** The patient understands and agrees to treatment.
■ **Implied:** Presumption that an unconscious or mentally incapacitated patient would, under normal circumstances, consent to life-saving treatment. *Note:* A competent adult who regains consciousness may refuse treatment.

- ■ **Expressed:** Verbal/nonverbal gesturing or written consent. *Note:* The absence of objection by a competent adult may be considered a form of expressed consent.
- ■ **Involuntary:** Consent to treat is granted by law enforcement.

Documentation: SOAP Format

Subjective Data
- ■ Chief complaint as described by patient
- ■ Family or bystander information
- ■ SAMPLE History
- ■ Symptom analysis (see OPQRST)

Objective Data
- ■ Initial impression of patient
- ■ Mechanism of injury
- ■ Vital signs and physical assessment

Assessment
- ■ Medical: Probable or suspected cause of medical problem (most often, patient's chief complaint)
- ■ Trauma: Obvious or suspected injury

Plan (including response to treatment)
- ■ Treatment (Oxygen, c-spine, intravenous drugs, drugs, splinting, etc.)
- ■ Patient response to treatment

Basic English to Spanish

English • [pro-**nun**-ci-**a**-tion] • *Spanish*

Introductions: Greetings

Hello [oh-lah] *Hola*

Good morning [bweh-nohs **dee**-ahs] *Buenos días*

Good afternoon [bweh-nohs tahr-dehs] *Buenos tardes*

Good evening [bweh-nahs **noh**-chehs] *Buenas noches*

My name is [meh yah-moh] *Me llamo*

I am a medic [soy el/lah **meh**-di-co/-ca] *Soy el/la médico(ca)*

I am a nurse [soy lah en-fehr-**meh**-ra] *Soy la enfermera*

What is your name? [koh-moh seh **yah**-mah oo-**stehd**] *¿Cómo se llama usted?*

How are you? [koh-moh eh-**stah** oo-**stehd**] *¿Cómo está usted?*

Very well [mwee b'**yehn**] *Muy bien*

Thank you [**grah**-s'yahs] *Gracias*

Yes, no [see, noh] *Sí, no*

Please [pohr fah-**vohr**] *Por favor*

You're welcome [deh **nah**-dah] *De nada*

Assessment: Areas of the Body

Head [kah-**beh**-sah] *Cabeza*

Eye [**oh**-hoh] *Ojo*

Ear [oh-**ee**-doh] *Oído*

Nose [nah-**rees**] *Nariz*

Throat [gahr-**gahn**-tah] *Garganta*

Neck [**kweh**-yoh] *Cuello*

Chest, heart [**peh**-choh, koh-rah-**sohn**] *Pecho, corazón*

Back [eh-**spahl**-dah] *Espalda*

Abdomen [ahb-doh-mehn] *Abdomen*
Stomach [eh-stoh-mah-goh] *Estómago*
Rectum [rehk-toh] *Recto*
Penis [peh-neh] *Pene*
Vagina [vah-hee-nah] *Vagina*
Arm [brah-soh] *Brazo*
Hand [mah-noh] *Mano*
Leg [p'yehr-nah] *Pierna*
Foot [p'yeh] *Pie*

Assessment: History

Do you have [T'yeh-neh oo-stehd] *¿Tiene usted?*
- **Difficulty breathing?** [di-fi-kul-**tad** pah-rah **res**-pee-rahr] *¿dificultad para respirar?*
- **Chest pain?** [doh-**lorh** en el **peh** cho] *¿dolor en el pecho?*
- **Abdominal pain?** [doh-**lorh** ab-do-mee-**nahl**] *¿dolor abdominal?*
- **Diabetes?** [dee-ah-**beh**-tehs] *¿diabetes?*

Are you [Ehs-**tah**] *¿Está?*
- **Dizzy?** [mar-eh-**ah**-do(da)] *¿mareado(da)?*
- **Nauseated?** [kohn **now**-say-as] *¿con nauseas?*
- **Pregnant?** [ehm-bah-rah-**sah**-dah] *¿embarazada?*

Are you allergic to any medications? [Ehs ah-**lehr**-hee-koh ah ahl-**goo**-nah meh-dee-**see**-nah] *¿Es alergico a alguna medicina?*

Assessment: Pain

Do you have pain? [T'yeh-neh oo-**stehd** doh-**lorh**?] *¿Tiene usted dolor?*
[(0) cero, (1) uno, (2) dos, (3) tres, (4) cuatro, (5) cinco, (6) seis, (7) siete, (8) ocho, (9) nueve, (10) diez]
Where does it hurt? [**Dohn**-deh leh **dweh**-leh] *¿Donde le duele?*
Is the pain [es oon doh-**lorh**] *¿Es un dolor?*
- **Dull?** [**leh**-veh] *¿leve?*
- **Aching?** [kan-**stan**-teh] *¿constante?*
- **Crushing?** [ah-plahs-**tahn**-teh] *¿aplastante?*

■ Sharp? [ah-**goo**-doh] *¿agudo?*

■ Stabbing? [ah-**poo**-nya-lahn-teh] *¿apuñalante?*

■ Burning? [ahr-**d'yen**-teh] *¿ardiente?*

Does it hurt when I press here? [Leh **dweh**-leh **kwahn**-doh leh ah-pree-**eh**-toh ah-**kee**] *¿Le duele cuando le aprieto aquí?*

Does it hurt to breathe deeply? [S'**yen**-teh oo-**stehd** doh-**lohr** kwahn-doh reh-**spee**-rah pro-foon-dah-**men**-teh] *¿Siente usted dolor cuando respira profundamente?*

Does it move to another area? [El doh-**lohr** seh moo-**eh**-veh a **oh**-tra ah-**reh**-ah] *¿El dolor se mueve a otra area?*

Is the pain better now? [Si-**en**-teh al-**goo**-nah me-**horr-i**-ah] *¿Siente alguna mejoria?*

Symbols and Abbreviations

ā before

α alpha

β beta

@ at

pound, quantity

" inch

® right

Ⓛ left

Ⓑ bilateral

↑ increase

↓ decrease

Ψ psychiatric

Ø none, no
Δ change
/ per, divided by
< less than
> greater than
° degrees
Rx treatment, prescription
μ micro
AAA abdominal aortic aneurysm
ABC automated blood count (airway, breathing, circulation)
ABD abdominal (dressing)
ABG arterial blood gas
AC before meals, antecubital
ACE angiotensin-converting enzyme
ACLS advanced cardiac life support
ACS acute coronary syndrome
ACTH adrenocorticotropic hormone
AD right ear
ADA American Diabetic Association
ADH antidiuretic hormone
ADHD attention deficit–hyperactivity disorder
ADL activities of daily living
ADR adverse drug reaction
AED automated external defibrillator
AHA American Heart Association
AIDS acquired immune deficiency syndrome
AKA above the knee amputation
ALOC altered level of consciousness
ALS advanced life support, amyotrophic lateral sclerosis
AMI acute myocardial infarction
AMS altered mental status, acute mountain sickness
AP anterior to posterior
APAP acetaminophen, Tylenol

APGAR appearance, pulse, grimace, activity, respiration
aPTT activated partial thromboplastin time
AS left ear
ASA aspirin (acetylsalicylic acid)
AU both ears
AV atrioventricular
AVB atrioventricular block
AVM arteriovenous malformation
AVPU alert, verbal, painful, unresponsive
BBB bundle branch block
BCC, BCCa basal cell carcinoma
BE barium enema, base excess
b.i.d. twice a day
BKA below the knee amputation
BM bowel movement
BMI body mass index
BP blood pressure
BPH benign prostatic hyperplasia
BPM beats per minute
BS blood sugar, bowel sounds
BSA body *or* burn surface area
BUN blood urea nitrogen
BVM bag-valve mask
c̄ with
°C degrees Celsius, centigrade
C&S, CS culture and sensitivity
Ca⁺⁺ calcium
CA cancer
CAD coronary artery disease
CBC complete blood count
CBG chemical blood glucose
CDC Centers for Disease Control
CF cystic fibrosis

CHB complete heart block

CHF congestive heart failure

CI cardiac index

Cl⁻ chloride

CNS central nervous system

CO carbon monoxide, cardiac output

CO₂ carbon dioxide

COPD chronic obstructive pulmonary disease

CP chest pain, cerebral palsy

CPAP continuous positive airway pressure

CPR cardiopulmonary resuscitation

CSF cerebrospinal fluid

CSM circulation, sensory, and motor

CT computed tomography

CV cardiovascular

CVA cerebrovascular accident

CVC central venous catheter

CVP central venous pressure

CX circumflex coronary artery

D₅W 5% dextrose in water

DBP diastolic BP

DC discontinue, direct current

DIC disseminated intravascular coagulopathy

DKA diabetic ketoacidosis

dL deciliter

DM diabetes mellitus

DOPE dislodgement, obstruction, pneumothorax, equipment

DT delirium tremors

DTS distance, time, shielding

DVT deep vein thrombosis

DZ, Dz disease

ECG, EKG electrocardiogram

ED erectile dysfunction, emergency department
EFM electronic fetal monitoring
EMS emergency medical services
EPS extrapyramidal symptoms
ESR erythrocyte sedimentation rate
ET endotracheal
EtOH alcohol
ETT endotracheal tube
°F degrees Fahrenheit
Fe iron
FFP fresh frozen plasma
FHR fetal heart rate
Fr, fr French
GCS Glasgow Coma Scale
GI gastrointestinal
gtt drop
GU genitourinary
H&H hemoglobin & hematocrit
h, hr hour
H$^+$ hydrogen ion
HA headache
HACE high altitude cerebral edema
HAPE high altitude pulmonary edema
HAZMAT hazardous material
HB heart block
HCl hydrogen chloride
HCO$_3$ carbonic acid
Hct hematocrit
HCTZ hydrochlorothiazide
HELLP hemolysis, elevated liver enzymes, low platelets
Hgb hemoglobin
HHNS hyperglycemic, hyperosmolar, nonketotic syndrome

HIV human immunodeficiency virus

HOB head of bed

HRT hormone replacement therapy

HS hour of sleep (night time)

HTN hypertension

HVS hyperventilation syndrome

IBC iron binding capacity

IBD irritable bowel disease

IBS irritable bowel syndrome

IBW ideal body weight

IC incident commander

ICP intracranial pressure

ICS intercostal space

ID intradermal

IDDM insulin-dependent diabetes mellitus

IHSS idiopathic hypertrophic subaortic stenosis

IM intramuscular

IN intranasal

INH isoniazid

INR international ratio

IO intraosseous

I/O intake & output

IV intravenous

IVC inferior vena cava

IVF IV fluid

IVP IV push

IVPB IV piggyback

J joule

JVD jugular vein distention

K+ potassium

KB knife blade (scalpel)

KCl potassium chloride

kg kilogram
LAD left anterior descending
LAT lateral
LBBB left bundle branch block
LLQ left lower quadrant
LMA laryngeal mask airway
LNMP last normal menstrual period
LOC level of consciousness
LPM liters per minute
LR lactated Ringer's
LTC left to count
LUQ left upper quadrant
mA milliampere
MAP mean arterial pressure
MAR medication administration record
MAST military antishock trousers
MCA motorcycle accident
mcg microgram
MCI mass casualty incident
MCL modified chest lead
mEq milliequivalent
mg milligram
Mg^{++} magnesium
MgSO$_4$ magnesium sulfate
MH malignant hyperthermia
MI myocardial infarction
min minute, minimum
mL milliliter
mm millimeter
mm Hg millimeter of mercury
MOA monoamine oxidase
MRI magnetic resonance imaging
MRSA methicillin-resistant *Staphylococcus aureus*

MS morphine, multiple sclerosis, musculoskeletal

MSO$_4$ morphine sulfate

MVA motor vehicle accident

Na$^+$ sodium

NAD no apparent/acute distress

NaHCO$_3$ sodium bicarbonate

NG nasogastric

NGT nasogastric tube

NI nasointestinal

NIDDM non-insulin-dependent diabetes mellitus

NPA nasopharyngeal airway

NPO nothing by mouth

NRB non-rebreather

NS normal saline

NSAID nonsteroidal anti-inflammatory drug

NSR normal sinus rhythm

NTG nitroglycerin

NTP nitroglycerin paste

n/v nausea and vomiting

O$_2$ oxygen

OCD obsessive compulsive disorder

OD overdose, right eye

OLMC online medical control

OPA oropharyngeal airway

OPP organophosphate

OPQRST onset, provocation, quality, radiation, severity, timing

OS left eye

OT occupational therapy

OTC over-the-counter

OU both eyes

oz ounce

p̄ after

PAC premature atrial complex

PAD peripheral artery disease

Pao_2 partial pressure of oxygen in arterial blood

PAP pulmonary artery pressure

PASG pneumatic anti-shock garment

PCI percutaneous intervention

PCW pulmonary capillary wedge pressure

PDA patent ductus arteriosus

PE pulmonary embolism/edema

PEA pulseless electrical activity

PEEP positive end-expiratory pressure

PERRL pupils equal, round, and reactive to light

PET positron emission tomography

PFIB perfluoroisobutene

pH potential of hydrogen

PICC peripherally inserted central catheter

PIH pregnancy-induced hypertension

PJC premature junctional complex

PMI point of maximal impulse

PMS premenstrual syndrome

PO by mouth, orally

PPD purified protein derivative (TB skin test)

PPE personal protective equipment

PPV positive-pressure ventilation

PPF plasma protein fraction

PRBC packed red blood cells

PRI PR interval

prn as needed

PSA prostate-specific antigen

PSI pounds per square inch

PSVT paroxysmal supraventricular tachycardia

Pt patient

PT prothrombin time, physical therapy

PTSD post-traumatic stress disorder

PTT partial thromboplastin time

PVC premature ventricular complex

PVD peripheral vascular disease

q, Q every

q.i.d. four times per day

q.o.d. every other day

R regular (insulin)

RA rheumatoid arthritis

RBBB right bundle branch block

RCA right coronary artery

RL Ringer's lactate

RLQ right lower quadrant

ROM range of motion, rupture of membranes

RR respiratory rate

RSI rapid sequence intubation

RSV respiratory syncytial virus

RT respiratory therapy, right

RTS revised trauma score

RUQ right upper quadrant

s̄ without

SAMPLE s/s, allergies, medications, pertinent history, last oral intake, events leading up

Sao$_2$ oxygen saturation

SBP systolic BP

SC, SQ subcutaneous

SCC squamous cell carcinoma

SI stroke index

SLP speech language pathology

SLUDGEM salivate, lacrimate, urinate, defecate, GI distress, emesis, meiosis or muscle twitching

SOB shortness of breath

Spo₂ pulse oximeter

ss, s/s signs and symptoms

STD sexually transmitted disease

SV stroke volume

SVC superior vena cava

SVR systemic venous resistance

T temperature

TB tuberculosis

TBSA total burn surface area

TCA tricyclic antidepressant

TCP transcutaneous pacing

TF tube feeding

TIA transient ischemic attack

t.i.d. three times per day

TKO to keep open

TPN total parenteral nutrition

TPR temperature, pulse, respirations

TVP transvenous pacing

u unit

UA urinalysis

UC ulcerative colitis

UO urine output

URI upper respiratory infection

UTI urinary tract infection

VAD vascular access device

VF ventricular fibrillation

VRE vancomycin-resistant *Enterococcus*

VRSA vancomycin-resistant *Staphylococcus aureus*

VT ventricular tachycardia

WBC white blood count

WC wheelchair

WPW Wolfe-Parkinson-White

COMMUNICATION WITH NONVERBAL PATIENT

Pain	1	2	3	4	5	6	7	8	9	10

Yes	No	Thank you

Cold	Hot	Sick

Thirsty	Hungry

Please Bring:
- Blanket
- Eyeglasses
- Dentures
- Hearing Aids

Empty:
- Bed pan
- Urinal
- Trash

Raise—Lower:
- Head
- Legs

Oral Care	Bath	Shower

TV	Lights	On	Off

Select References and Web Resources

GENERAL

Centers for Disease Control and Prevention (CDC) http://www.cdc.gov/

CDC *Travelers' Health—Yellow Book: HEPATITIS B* http://wwwnc.cdc
.gov/travel/yellowbook/2010/chapter-2/hepatitis-b.aspx#849

Central Intelligence Agency https://www.cia.gov

Diversity, Healing, and Health Care

http://www.gasi-ves.org/diversity.htm

Countries and Their Cultures http://www.everyculture.com

Food and Agriculture Organization of the United Nations/*Nutrition Country
Profiles*

http://www.fao.org/ag/agn/nutrition/profiles_en.stm

International Business Etiquette http://www.cyborlink.com/

La Leche League International *Center for Breastfeeding Information*
http://www.llli.org/cbi/bfstats03.html

Travel Etiquette http://www.traveletiquette.co.uk

UN Data http://data.un.org/

Prevalence of obesity among adults
http://data.un.org/Data.aspx?q=prevalence&d=GenderStat&f=
inID%3A43

UNICEF *United Nations Special Sessions on Children* (8–10 May 2002)
http://www.unicef.org/specialsession/about/sg-report.htm

UNICEF *Statistics—Child Malnutrition*
http://www.unicef.org/specialsession/about/sgreport-pdf/02_
ChildMalnutrition_D7341Insert_English.pdf

World Health Organization (WHO) http://www.who.int/en/

WHO *Mental Health Atlas 2005*
http://www.who.int/mental_health/evidence/mhatlas05/en/index.html

World Sites Atlas *HIV/AIDS Adult Prevalence Rate*
http://www.sitesatlas.com/Thematic-Maps/
    HIV-AIDS-adult-prevalence-rate.html

Wrong Diagnosis *Statistics by Country for Alcoholism*
http://www.wrongdiagnosis.com/a/alcoholism/stats-country.htm

COUNTRY-SPECIFIC

Stanford University *Health and Health Care of American Indian and Alaska Native Elders*
http://www.stanford.edu/group/ethnoger/americanindian.html

Colombia Reports *1.6 Million Children in Colombia Perform Child Labor*
    http://colombiareports.com/colombia-news/news/4512-16-million-
    children-in-colombia-work.html

Friedman School of Nutrition Science and Policy, Tufts University *Atlas of Hunger and Malnutrition in the Dominican Republic*
http://nutrition.tufts.edu/docs/pdf/fpan/DR_Report_Final.pdf

MedIndia http://www.medindia.net/

MedIndia *Lifestyle and Wellness: Teen Pregnancy*
http://www.medindia.net/news/lifestyleandwellness/Teen-Pregnancy-
    34940-1.htm

Pan American Health Organization http://www.paho.org

BBC News *Smoking Curbs: The Global Picture: Europe* (1 July 2009)
    http://news.bbc.co.uk/2/hi/3758707.stm#ouropе

allAfrica.com *Nigeria: Obesity, Diabetes Epidemics Loom*
http://allafrica.com/stories/200810310616.html

United Nations Office on Drugs and Crime *Nigeria Country Profile*
    http://www.unodc.org/nigeria/en/abuse.html

University of Kuopio, Finland *Antenatal Care and Maternal Mortality in Nigeria*
http://www.uku.fi/kansy/eng/antenal_care_nigeria.pdf

Motherland Nigeria http://www.motherlandnigeria.com/life.html

The New York Times: Europe *Cigarettes: Killing Russia Softly*
http://www.nytimes.com/2008/09/07/world/europe/07iht-smoking
.4.15954384.html?_r=1

BBC News *Russia's Mental Health Revolution* (28 June 2003)
http://news.bbc.co.uk/2/hi/health/3026648.stm

University of Miami Comprehensive Drug Research Center *Substance Abuse and HIV in Russia*

cdrc.med.miami.edu/documents/DRUGS%20IN%20RUSSIA-final.ppt

Culture Crossing *Uganda*

http://www.culturecrossing.net/basics_business_student_details.php
?Id=13&CID=212

BOOKS

1. Andrews, A.M. & Boyle, J.S. (2003) *Transcultural Concepts in Nursing Care*.
2. Bennett, M.J. (Ed.) (1998) *Basic Concepts of Intercultural Communication*, Yarmouth, Maine, Intercultural Press.
3. Bigby, J. (Ed.) (2003) *Cross Cultural Medicine*, Philadelphia, American College of Physicians.
4. D'Avanzo, C.E. & Geissler, E.M. (2003) *Cultural Health Assessment Pocket Guide Series*, 4th ed., St. Louis, Mosby.
5. Davis-Floyd, R.E. & Sargent, C.F. (Eds.) (1997) *Childbirth and Authoritative Knowledge*, Berkeley, University of California Press.
6. Dresser, N. (1996) *Multicultural Manners*, New York, John Wiley & Sons.
7. Finkler, K. (1994) *Women in Pain: Gender and Morbidity in Mexico*, Philadelphia, University of Pennsylvania Press.
8. Foster, G.M. & Anderson, B.G. (1978) *Medical Anthropology*, New York, Alfred A. Knopf.
9. Gaby, A.R. (Ed.) (2006) *A–Z Guide to Drug-Herb-Vitamin Interactions*, New York, Three Rivers Press.
10. Galanti, G. (2004) *Caring for Patients From Different Cultures*, 3rd ed., Philadelphia, University of Pennsylvania Press.

11. Hill, P. & Lipson, J.G. (2003) *Caring for Women Cross-Culturally*, Philadelphia, F.A. Davis.

12. Kirkwood, N.A. (1993) *A Hospital Handbook on Multiculturalism and Religion*, Harrisburg, Morehouse Publishing.

13. Lassiter, S.M. (1995) *Multicultural Clients: A Professional Handbook for Health Care Providers and Social Workers*. Westport, Conn., Greenwood Press

14. Leininger, M. & McFarland, M.R. (2002) *Transcultural Nursing: Concepts, Theories, Research and Practice*, 3rd ed., New York, McGraw-Hill, Medical Publishing Division.

15. Lipson, J.C. & Dibble, S.L. (1996) *Culture & Nursing Care: A Pocket Guide*, San Francisco, UCSF Nursing Press.

16. Lipson, J.G. & Steiger, N.J. (1996) *Self-Care Nursing in a Multicultural Context*, Thousand Oaks, Calif., Sage Productions.

17. Morrison, T. & Conaway, W.A. (1994) *Kiss, Bow, or Shake Hands*, Massachusetts, Adams Media Corp.

18. Munoz C. & Hilgenberg C. "Ethnopharmacology." American Journal of Nursing 2005;105(8)40–48.

19. Munoz, C. & Luckmann, J. (2005) *Transcultural Communication in Nursing*, 2nd ed., Australia, Thomson Publisher.

20. Myers, E. (2001) North American Nursing Diagnosis. *RN Notes*, per Taber's Cyclopedic Medical Dictionary, ed. 19., FA Davis, Philadelphia.

21. Powell, M. (2004) *Behave Yourself! The Essential Guide to International Etiquette*, Philadephia, Globe Pequot Press.

22. Rundle, A. & Carvalho, M. (1999) *Cultural Competence in Health Care: A Practical Guide*, San Francisco, Jossey-Bass.

23. Spector, R.E. (2000) *Cultural Care: Guidelines to Heritage Assessment and Health Traditions*, Upper Saddle River, New Jersey, Prentice Hall.

24. The World Factbook at www.cia/gov/cia/publications/factbook/fields/2122.html

Index

Pocket Guide to Culturally Sensitive Health Care

Barbara Stuart
Catherine Cherry • Jill Stuart

How much eye contact does my patient expect and accept from me?

Are there certain foods that are forbidden in this culture?

Are any specific diseases prevalent in my patient's native country?

Take the guessing out of assessing!
Increase your knowledge, awareness, and sensitivity to the 25 cultures most commonly seen in clinical settings.

Comprehensive and evidence-based
For each culture, you'll find information on the 11 areas of care most discussed by health-care professionals with their clients.

- Communication
- Nutrition
- Physical illness
- Mental illness
- Sexuality
- Pain
- Childbearing
- Child rearing
- Family role
- Spirituality and beliefs
- Death and dying

Provide safer, more personalized care for your culturally diverse patients!

F.A. DAVIS COMPANY

Independent Publishers Since 1879
www.fadavis.com

ISBN 13: 978-0-8036-2263-0

9 780803 622630